Viruses Associated with Gastroenteritis

Viruses Associated with Gastroenteritis

Guest Editors

Celso Cunha
Claudia Istrate

MDPI

Basel • Beijing • Wuhan • Barcelona • Belgrade • Novi Sad • Cluj • Manchester

Guest Editors
Celso Cunha
Institute of Hygiene and
Tropical Medicine
NOVA University
Lisbon
Portugal

Claudia Istrate
Faculty of Veterinary
Medicine
University of Lisbon
Lisbon
Portugal

Editorial Office
MDPI AG
Grosspeteranlage 5
4052 Basel, Switzerland

This is a reprint of the Special Issue, published open access by the journal *Viruses* (ISSN 1999-4915), freely accessible at: https://www.mdpi.com/journal/viruses/special_issues/5I99946KTW.

For citation purposes, cite each article independently as indicated on the article page online and as indicated below:

Lastname, A.A.; Lastname, B.B. Article Title. *Journal Name* **Year**, *Volume Number*, Page Range.

ISBN 978-3-7258-8365-3 (Hbk)
ISBN 978-3-7258-8366-0 (PDF)
https://doi.org/10.3390/books978-3-7258-8366-0

Contents

About the Editors

Celso Cunha

Celso Cunha is professor of Virology and the Director of the Medical Microbiology Unit of the Institute of Hygiene and Tropical Medicine, NOVA University Lisbon. He holds a PhD in Biology from University of Lisbon (1992), and was awarded a Habilitation title in Medical Microbiology from NOVA University of Lisbon (2012). His career has been dedicated to the study of different aspects of infection, replication, host–pathogen interactions, and molecular epidemiology of several viruses, including African swine fever virus, Hepatitis B virus, Hepatitis D virus, HIV, and Rotavirus. He has supervised 10 PhD thesis and coordinated 7 projects financed by national and international agencies. Celso Cunha has published 50 manuscripts in peer-reviewed indexed journals, is the coauthor of book chapters, and holds 2 patents. He has acted as the evaluator of project proposals for 12 international and 2 national funding agencies and as a reviewer for over 40 different indexed international journals. He was member of the Editorial Board of 3 international indexed journals. He has a pedagogic career lasting more than 25 years at the master's and PhD levels and coordinated a master's program in Biomedical Sciences. During his scientific and pedagogic career, he has been awarded several prizes, including the Public Health and Microbiology Prizes awarded by the National Institute of Health in Portugal.

Claudia Istrate

Claudia Istrate is a veterinarian and researcher acting as external collaborator for the Centre for Interdisciplinary Research in Animal Health, a research centre of the University of Lisbon in Portugal. She holds a PhD in Biology from NOVA University of Lisbon (2007), time when started working on the development of an alternative rotavirus vaccine based on virus-like particles produced through recombinant DNA technology. Since then, she continued working on several projects: 1). Molecular epidemiology of viruses causing acute gastroenteritis (AGE) in Portugal and Portuguese-speaking countries, with emphasis on rotavirus and norovirus, which are both viruses with high impact on public health and scarce data from the locations mentioned above 2). Host genetic factors (i.e., human blood group antigens) associated with individual susceptibility to these viral diseases and their relationship with rotavirus vaccine efficacy. 3). Zoonotic and veterinary viruses with great impact on animal health (i.e., African swine fever virus). Claudia has coordinated 10 research projects funded by national and international agencies and has published 24 publications: 20 international peer-reviewed publications, 1 article citing African studies, 1 book chapter, and 3 publications in national journals. She has also presented her research at approximately 50 national and international congresses. She has received several grants to attend professional courses and conferences, being invited to present her research internationally (orally and in poster sessions). Finally, she has organized science outreach activities for professionals and the general public.

viruses

MDPI

Editorial

Special Issue: "Viruses Associated with Gastroenteritis"

Celso Cunha [1,*] and Claudia Istrate [2]

1 Global Health and Tropical Medicine (GHTM), Institute of Hygiene and Tropical Medicine (IHMT-NOVA), NOVA University, Rua da Junqueira, 100, 1349-008 Lisbon, Portugal
2 Interdisciplinary Center for Research in Animal Health (CIISA), Faculty of Veterinary Medicine, University of Lisbon, 1300-477 Lisbon, Portugal; claudiaistrate@fmv.ulisboa.pt
* Correspondence: ccunha@ihmt.unl.pt

1. Introduction

Diarrheal diseases are the third leading cause of death in children under 5 years of age, with approximately 450.000 deaths per year, especially in low and middle income countries (LMICs). Yet, the burden of acute gastroenteritis (AGE) can be significantly reduced by vaccination campaigns and implementation of simple preventive sanitation measures. Despite the availability of four vaccines pre-qualified by WHO, of which two are recommended to be introduced in national immunization programs worldwide since 2009, rotaviruses remain the main cause of AGE with the highest burden in African sub-Saharan countries. Rotaviruses and noroviruses account for about two thirds of deaths caused by diarrhea in children under 5 years of age. However, other viruses, namely adenoviruses, sapoviruses, and astroviruses, may also have a non-negligible impact.

This Special Issue includes eight articles. The majority reports new data on the molecular epidemiology and genome evolution of rotavirus, norovirus, adenovirus, and sapovirus. Overall, the authors highlight the need for the implementation of full genome surveillance programs, continuous monitoring of emergence of new variants and strains, and their potential impact on the efficacy of currently available vaccines and influence on the design of future formulations.

2. Contributions

Vita et al. [1] present new data on the status, evolution and molecular epidemiology of rotaviruses in Angola (2021–2022), a country where epidemiological data is scarce, namely in the period after vaccine introduction, in 2014. In Brazil, Silva et al. [2] conducted a retrospective study (2012–2014) highlighting the emergence of new multiple reassortment events with rotaviruses commonly found in other continents, namely Africa and Asia. The detection of new variants and strains with potential to replace those currently circulating is stressed in both studies.

The importance of sustained genotyping and phylogenetic analysis of new isolates is also underlined for noroviruses. In Finland (2024/2025), Al-Hello et al. [3] report widespread high rates of detection of GII strains that cluster with other GII strains earlier detected in Europe and the United States. Moreover, Lee et al. [4] assessed norovirus detection rates in pre- and post-COVID-19 pandemic periods (2019–2024) in Korea. The most commonly found strains were also GII. However, a shifting genotype dynamic was detected in 2024. Both studies underscore the need for continuous surveillance with added importance in the context of norovirus vaccine development, and reinforcement of public health interventions.

The impact of high levels of expression of bacterial lipopolysaccharide (LPS) genes on norovirus infection was investigated in South Africa (2018–2020) by Kgosana et al. [5]. A positive correlation was found between high levels of expression of LPS and development of norovirus diarrhea in children aged between 3.5 and 9 months old. This observation may suggest an eventual role of bacterial LPSs and perhaps other components of the microbiome in the course and outcome of norovirus infections. This hypothesis deserves more comprehensive attention in a broader context of viral infections of the gastrointestinal tract.

The importance of monitoring circulating variants is further underlined for human enteric adenoviruses in a retrospective study conducted by Mello et al. [6] in Brazil (2021–2023). Sequencing of the hexon and/or fiber genes revealed that HAdV-F40/41 was the most frequently detected human enteric adenovirus genotype in stool samples from AGE cases. This genotype was also associated with higher viral loads when compared to non-enteric HAdVs.

Sapoviruses were investigated in a study by Guo et al. [7] using samples obtained from a viral diarrhea surveillance network in China (2022–2023). The overall detection rate was higher in children under 5 years of age (2.37%). Eight genotypes were identified by sequencing with the highest variation rates observed in the NS1 region of the genome.

At last, the work by Luchs et al. [8] spotlights an overlap of respiratory and enteric syndromes in children $\leq$ 3 years of age, in Brazil (2021). A search for different viruses was performed in 20 paired swab and stool samples from children with diarrheal and respiratory symptoms allowing detecting seven different virus families that may cause respiratory and enteric diseases: Human bocavirus, Norovirus, Human enteric adenovirus, Parechovirus, Enterovirus, Respiratory syncytial virus, and Influenza A virus. Human bocaviruses, which have been previously associated with both AGE and respiratory diseases, and noroviruses, were detected in 75% of cases, with co-infections observed in 65% of patients. Although limited by the small number of enrolled patients, the study points to the importance of implementation of accurate differential diagnosis procedures.

3. Outlook and Final Remarks

The burden of AGE remains unacceptably high, namely in children living in LMICs. Simple, and often low-cost sanitation measures, like provision of universal access to drinking water as well as the implementation of effective campaigns designed to improve hygiene and health literacy have a proven significant positive impact. Yet, these interventions should go hand in hand with effective vaccination campaigns. Apart from the aforementioned vaccines against rotaviruses, there are currently at least three norovirus vaccine candidates in different stages of development: a virus-like particle (VLP) formulation, a bivalent oral vaccine, and a trivalent mRNA vaccine. Even so, development of new and more effective formulations is only one of the many challenges that we face to reduce the burden of AGE. Raising awareness among policy decision makers for the urgent need to implement effective surveillance plans and preventive strategies is of utmost importance. The contributions contained in this Special Issue are certainly a drop in the ocean but the ocean continues to rise.

We thank all authors for sharing their high quality and impactful research as well as the reviewers whose selfless work were fundamental to maintaining scientific rigor and improved the quality of manuscripts. Finally, we express sincere gratitude to all members of the editorial staff for their commitment and professionalism since the beginning of the preparation of the Special Issue.

Author Contributions: Writing, review and editing, C.C. and C.I. All authors have read and agreed to the published version of the manuscript.

Conflicts of Interest: The authors declare no conflicts of interest.

References

1. Vita, D.G.; Santiso-Bellón, C.; Lemos, M.; Neto, Z.; Fortes-Gabriel, E.; Brito, M.; Sebastião, C.S.; Rodriguez-Diaz, J.; Cunha, C.; Istrate, C. *Rotavirus alphagastroenteritidis*: Circulating Strains After the Introduction of the Rotavirus Vaccine (Rotarix®) in Luanda Province of Angola. *Viruses* **2025**, *17*, 858. [CrossRef] [PubMed]
2. Silva, V.C.M.; França, Y.; Azevedo, L.S.d.; Guiducci, R.; Villela, E.F.d.M.; Luchs, A. Unveiling the Genomic Landscape of G2P[6] Rotavirus a Strains in Brazil: Evolutionary and Epidemiological Perspectives. *Viruses* **2025**, *17*, 1103. [CrossRef] [PubMed]
3. Al-Hello, H.; Rimhanen-Finne, R.; Savolainen-Kopra, C. Delayed Emergence of Norovirus GII.17 in Finland: Foodborne Outbreaks Reported During the 2024/25 Season. *Viruses* **2025**, *17*, 1530. [CrossRef]
4. Lee, M.; Cho, S.-R.; Jo, Y.; Lee, D.-Y.; Han, M.-G.; Park, S.-W. Trends in Norovirus Genotypes in South Korea, 2019–2024: Insights from Nationwide Dual Typing Surveillance. *Viruses* **2025**, *17*, 1572. [CrossRef]
5. Kgosana, L.P.; Seheri, M.L.; Magwira, C.A. Significant Association Between Increased Abundance of Selected Bacterial Lipopolysaccharides and Norovirus Diarrhea Among South African Infants. *Viruses* **2025**, *17*, 278. [CrossRef] [PubMed]
6. Mello, M.d.S.; Malta, F.C.; Fialho, A.M.; Burlandy, F.M.; Fumian, T.M. Molecular Epidemiology of Human Adenovirus from Acute Gastroenteritis Cases in Brazil After the COVID-19 Pandemic Period, 2021–2023. *Viruses* **2025**, *17*, 577. [CrossRef] [PubMed]
7. Guo, M.; Li, M.; Liu, T.; Sun, W.; Du, K.; Yang, S.; Fu, Z.; Kou, Z. Epidemiological and Genetic Characteristics of Sapovirus in Shandong, China, 2022–2023. *Viruses* **2025**, *17*, 469. [CrossRef] [PubMed]
8. Luchs, A.; Adiwardana, N.S.; Rocha, L.C.d.; Viana, E.; Guadagnucci, S.; Parise, A.; Silva, V.C.M.; Azevedo, L.S.d.; Guiducci, R.; França, Y.; et al. Concurrent Circulation of Viral Agents in Pediatric Patients Presenting with Respiratory Illness and Diarrheal Symptoms in Metropolitan Region of São Paulo, Brazil, 2021. *Viruses* **2025**, *17*, 497. [CrossRef] [PubMed]

https://doi.org/10.3390/v18010022

viruses

MDPI

Article

Concurrent Circulation of Viral Agents in Pediatric Patients Presenting with Respiratory Illness and Diarrheal Symptoms in Metropolitan Region of São Paulo, Brazil, 2021

Adriana Luchs [1,2,*], Natanael Sutikno Adiwardana [3], Leonardo Cecilio da Rocha [2], Ellen Viana [1], Simone Guadagnucci [1], Adriana Parise [1], Vanessa Cristina Martins Silva [1], Lais Sampaio de Azevedo [1], Raquel Guiducci [1], Yasmin França [1], Natacha Luana Pezzuol Frank [3], Ana Lucia Nascimento da Silva [3], Andre Luiz Vianna de Oliveira [4], André Henrique Souza Azevedo [4], Bárbara Segatelli Carreteiro [4] and Maurício Lacerda Nogueira [2,5]

1 Virology Center, Adolfo Lutz Institute, Sao Paulo 01246-902, Brazil
2 São José do Rio Preto School of Medicine (FAMERP), São José do Rio Preto 15090-000, Brazil; mauricio.nogueira@edu.famerp.br (M.L.N.)
3 Infection Prevention and Control Service, Barueri Central Emergency Center, Barueri 06401-000, Brazil; nateldiw@yahoo.com.br (N.S.A.)
4 Pediatric Emergency Care, Barueri Central Emergency Center (SAMEB), Barueri 06401-000, Brazil
5 Department of Pathology, University of Texas Medical Branch, Galveston, TX 7555-0609, USA
* Correspondence: driluchs@gmail.com or adriana.luchs@ial.sp.gov.br; Tel.: +55-11-3068-2909

Abstract: Pneumonia and diarrhea are the leading causes of death in children under 5 globally, worsened by viral infections. This study investigates viral agents in children $\leq$ 3 years with respiratory illness and diarrhea in Metropolitan Region of São Paulo, Brazil, during spring 2021. Twenty paired samples (oropharyngeal swab and feces) were tested using in-house qPCR for HBoV and HAdV, RT-qPCR for RVA, EV, PeV-A, and NoV, and a commercial RT-qPCR kit for SARS-CoV-2, Flu A/B, and RSV. HAstV was detected with conventional nested (RT)-PCR. Positive samples were sequenced for molecular characterization and phylogenetic analysis. Seven viruses were identified: HBoV, NoV, HAdV, PeV-A, EV, RSV, and Flu A. HBoV and NoV were detected in 75% of cases, with co-infection in 65% of patients, indicating their involvement in the gastro-respiratory illness. Genotyping of HBoV (HBoV-1), NoV (GII.4_Sydney[P16], GII.2[P16], and GII.4_Sydney[P31]), EV (Coxsackievirus A6), HAdV (species C, type 6), and PeV-A (genotype 1) showed local virus diversity. Phylogenetic analysis indicated no ongoing community outbreak, with distinct clusters observed. The findings highlight the overlap of respiratory and enteric diseases, revealing local viral diversity and high exposure to enteric viruses. This underscores the challenges in differential diagnosis and the need for syndromic surveillance.

Keywords: viral infections; gastro-respiratory illness; co-infection; syndromic surveillance; viral diversity

1. Introduction

Pneumonia and diarrhea are leading causes of death in children under age 5 worldwide, resulting in 1.23 million annual fatalities (https://www.jhsph.edu/ivac/wp-content/uploads/2020/11/IVAC_PDPR_2020.pdf accessed on 28 February 2025). Viral infections causing diarrhea have posed a significant public health challenge over decades, yet clinical presentations often lack clear indications of specific viral agents [1]. Group A rotaviruses

(RVA), noroviruses (NoV), enteric adenoviruses (HAdV), and astroviruses (HAstV) are commonly identified as enteric viral pathogens in cases of acute gastroenteritis [1].

Gastrointestinal symptoms are also observed in various respiratory virus infections, such as influenza and severe acute respiratory syndrome coronavirus 2 (SARS-CoV-2) [2]. These symptoms may arise due to co-infections involving respiratory and enteric viruses during concurrent outbreaks of respiratory infections and gastroenteritis, potentially linking symptoms that could mislead clinical assessments [3]. Enteroviruses (EVs) are widely associated with respiratory diseases, acute flaccid paralysis, aseptic meningitis, encephalitis, hand-foot-and-mouth disease, febrile illnesses, neonatal sepsis, and cardiopathies [4]. While EVs have been sporadically linked to diarrhea in some studies, their definitive role in causing human gastroenteritis remains uncertain [5]. Emerging viruses like human bocaviruses (HBoV) and Parechoviruses A (PeV-A) have also been reported to be associated with both acute gastroenteritis and respiratory diseases [6,7].

Surveillance is crucial for public health, providing essential data for guiding interventions. However, there remains a lack of comprehensive data on the syndromic landscape of viral agents associated with respiratory and diarrheal illnesses in Brazil. Most studies have focused primarily on diagnosing single viral infections (e.g., RVA or NoV) in cases of acute diarrhea or specific viruses such as Influenza A/B (Flu A/B), SARS-CoV-2, and Respiratory Syncytial Virus (RSV) in investigations of Severe Acute Respiratory Illness [8,9]. Implementing syndromic surveillance that includes testing for newly emerging viruses could enhance understanding of the spectrum of viral agents linked to acute gastroenteritis and respiratory diseases in Brazil. This approach could particularly advance differential diagnosis in cases presenting with combined gastrointestinal and respiratory symptoms.

In this study, we identified and molecularly characterized viral agents causing acute respiratory disease in children $\leq$ 3 years old presenting with diarrheic symptoms in the northwestern region of the Metropolitan Region of São Paulo, Brazil, during spring 2021. Phylogenetic analysis was conducted to explore genetic relationships with previously reported viruses.

2. Material and Methods

2.1. Study Population

A significant increase in children under 3 years of age presenting with both respiratory and gastrointestinal symptoms was noted at the Pediatric Emergency Care unit of Barueri Medical Assistance Service (SAMEB) in mid-August 2021. With negative COVID-19 tests, the possibility of an emerging virus (e.g., HBoV or PeV-A) was considered. Therefore, the present study included children with enteric and respiratory symptoms whose parents provided the Informed Consent Form. After three months, recruitment was halted as the number of cases decreased. It is important to highlight that limited staff availability in the overwhelmed COVID-19 emergency room hindered further recruitment.

This case report was conducted from August 30th to December 6th, 2021, involving 20 children aged $\leq$ 3 years who presented with respiratory and diarrheic symptoms at SAMEB. The study utilized secondary data from medical records collected during routine care, ensuring patient confidentiality through the anonymization of all information. Basic demographic details (age, gender) and clinical information (symptom onset and collection dates, symptoms like cough, diarrhea, vomiting, fever, and runny nose) were extracted from clinical records (Table 1).

Table 1. Clinical and demographic data from the 20 children with acute respiratory disease and diarrheic symptoms, Barueri, São Paulo, Brazil, spring 2021.

ID	Gender	Age	Onset Date	Collection Date	City	Signs and Symptoms	HBoV, Type	RVA	HAdV, Type	EV, Type	SARS-CoV-2	Flu A/B	RSV	HAstV	NoV, Group	NoV Strain	PeV-A, Type	Sample
N01	Male	1 year	August 8	August 30	Barueri	Diarrhea	+, NT	-	-	-	-	-	+	-	-		-	Swab
							-	-	-	-	-	-	+	-	+, GII	GII.4 Sydney[P16]	-	Feces
N02	Male	1 year	August 28	September 3	Barueri	Diarrhea, vomiting, coryza, cough, fever	+, NT	-	-	-	-	-	-	-	-		-	Swab
							-	-	-	-	-	-	-	-	+, GII	GII.4 Sydney[P16]	-	Feces
N03	Female	1 year	August 31	September 3	Carapicuiba	Diarrhea	+, NT	-	-	-	-	-	+	-	-		-	Swab
							+, NT	-	-	-	-	-	-	-	+, GII	NT	-	Feces
N04	Male	2 years	September 5	September 5	Barueri	Diarrhea, vomiting	+, HBoV-1	-	-	+, CVA6	-	-	-	-	-		-	Swab
							+, HBoV-1	-	-	+, CVA6	-	-	-	-	+, GII	GII.4 Sydney[P31]	-	Feces
N05	Female	1 year	September 5	September 6	Osasco	Diarrhea, cough, fever	+, HBoV-1	-	-	-	-	-	-	-	-		-	Swab
							+, HBoV-1	-	-	-	-	-	-	-	+, GII	GII.2[P16]	-	Feces
N06	Female	6 months	September 6	September 8	Osasco	Diarrhea, cough, vomiting	-	-	-	-	-	-	-	-	+, GII	GII.4 Sydney[P16]	+, NT	Feces
N07	Female	1 year	September 9	September 10	Barueri	Diarrhea	+, HBoV-1	-	-	-	-	-	-	-	+, GII	GII.4 Sydney[P16]	-	Feces
N08	Male	2 years	September 12	September 13	Barueri	Diarrhea, vomiting, coryza, fever, productive cough, abdominal pain	+, HBoV-1	-	-	-	-	-	-	-	+, GII	NT	-	Feces
N09	Male	3 years	September 20	September 21	Barueri	Diarrhea, vomiting	-	-	-	-	-	-	-	-	-		-	Swab
							+, NT	-	-	-	-	-	-	-	+, GII	GII.2[P16]	-	Feces
N10	Male	20 days	September 18	September 21	Barueri	Vomiting, fever	+, HBoV-1	-	-	-	-	-	-	-	-		-	Swab
							+, NT	-	-	-	-	-	-	-	-		-	Feces
N11	Female	1 year	September 12	September 13	Carapicuiba	Diarrhea, vomiting, coryza, cough, fever	-	-	-	-	-	-	-	-	-		-	Swab
							+, HBoV-1	-	+, C6	-	-	-	-	-	+, GII	GII.4 Sydney[P16]	-	Feces
N12	Male	2 years	September 20	September 22	Barueri	Diarrhea, vomiting, coryza, sore throat, abdominal pain	+, HBoV-1	-	-	-	-	-	-	-	-		-	Swab
							+, NT	-	-	-	-	-	-	-	+, GII	GII.4 Sydney[P16]	-	Feces
N13	Male	11 days	September 20	September 21	Barueri	Fever	+, NT	-	-	-	-	-	-	-	-		-	Swab
							+, NT	-	-	-	-	-	-	-	-		-	Feces
N14	Female	6 months	September 26	September 28	Carapicuiba	Diarrhea, cough	-	-	-	-	-	-	-	-	-		-	Swab
							-	-	-	-	-	-	-	-	-		-	Feces
N15	Male	1 year	October 2	October 8	Sao Paulo	Diarrhea, vomiting, coryza, fever, sneeze, productive cough, abdominal pain	+, HBoV-1	-	+, C6	-	-	-	-	-	-		-	Swab
							+, NT	-	-	-	-	-	-	-	+, GII	GII.2[P16]	-	Feces
N16	Female	1 year	October 7	October 9	Barueri	Diarrhea, Fever	+, NT	-	-	-	-	-	-	-	-		-	Swab
							+, NT	-	-	-	-	-	-	-	+, GII	GII.4 Sydney[P16]	-	Feces
N17	Female	5 months	October 11	October 11	Osasco	Diarrhea, vomiting	-	-	-	+, CVA6	-	-	-	-	-		-	Swab
							-	-	-	+, CVA6	-	-	-	-	+, GII	GII.4 Sydney[P16]	+, PeV-A1	Feces
N18	Male	1 year	October 14	October 17	Carapicuiba	Diarrhea, vomiting, coryza, sneeze, productive cough	+, NT	-	-	-	-	-	-	-	-		-	Swab
							-	-	-	-	-	-	-	-	+, GII	GII.4 Sydney[P16]	-	Feces
N19	Male	1 year	November 30	December 4	Itapevi	Diarrhea, coryza, productive cough, fever	-	-	-	-	-	-	-	-	-		-	Swab
							-	-	-	-	-	-	-	-	-		-	Feces
N20	Male	2 years	December 2	December 6	Carapicuiba	Diarrhea, vomiting, coryza, cough	-	-	-	-	-	Flu A	-	-	-		-	Swab
							-	-	-	-	-	-	-	-	-		-	Feces

NT: non-typed.

Oropharyngeal swabs and fecal samples collected from each patient were stored at −20 °C and later screened for viruses at the Research Laboratory of Virology, Faculty of Medicine of São José do Rio Preto (FAMERP). SAMEB, affiliated with the Municipality of Barueri's Health Department, operates under Brazil's Unified Health System (Sistema Único de Saúde—SUS) and serves as a key healthcare facility in the northwest region of São Paulo municipality, Brazil. Barueri is ranked as the 14th wealthiest city in Brazil, with a population of 316,473 residents spread over 65.70 km^2 (https://www.ibge.gov.br/cidades-e-estados/sp/barueri.html accessed on 28 February 2025).

2.2. Viral Screening

Viral DNA/RNA from oropharyngeal and 10% fecal samples was extracted using the Zymo Quick-DNA/RNATM Viral MagBead kit (Zymo Research®, Orange, CA, USA) following the manufacturer's instructions. Screening for RVA, EV, NoV, and PeV-A utilized reverse transcription quantitative real-time PCR (RT-qPCR) with established primers and protocols [10–13]. HAdV and HBoV detection employed quantitative real-time PCR (qPCR) as described by Heim et al. [14] and Lu et al. [15], respectively. SARS-CoV-2, Flu A, Flu B, and RSV were detected using the Allplex™ SARS-CoV-2/FluA/FluB/RSV RT-qPCR kit (Seegene Inc., Seoul, Republic of Korea) following manufacturer guidelines. Samples were considered positive at Ct values $\leq$ 39. Reverse transcription used random primers, and HAstV detection in cDNA employed heminested PCR targeting the RdRp gene (422 bp) with protocols by Chu et al. [16].

2.3. HAdV, HBoV, NoV, EV, and PeV-A Typing

Positive HAdV, HBoV, EV, NoV, and PeV-A samples underwent molecular characterization. Viral DNA/RNA from oropharyngeal swabs and/or feces was directly amplified and sequenced using Sanger sequencing for phylogenetic analysis.

HAdV strains were genotyped using hexon gene-specific primers (Ad1 and Ad2) targeting a 482-bp section, following Xu et al.'s protocol [17]. HBoV samples were amplified using VP1/VP2 region-specific primers in a conventional PCR method by Durigon et al. [18], yielding a 657-bp amplicon.

NoV samples were amplified using MON 431 and G2SKR primers targeting a 570-bp fragment covering regions B and C (3′-end of ORF1 and 5′-end of ORF2) [19] with the SuperScript III One-Step RT-PCR System (Invitrogen, Life Technologies, Carlsbad, CA, USA).

EV and PeV-A samples underwent conventional RT-PCR with random primers. EV VP1 region-specific primers were used in a semi-nested PCR following Iturriza-Cómara et al.'s method [20], while PeV-A samples were amplified using nested PCR targeting the VP3/VP1 junction region according to Ghanem-Zoubi et al.'s procedure [21].

PCR products were analyzed on 1.5% agarose gel with GelRed™ and a 100-bp molecular size ladder. Sequencing was performed using the BigDye™ Kit v3.1 (Applied Biosystems, Foster City, CA, USA) and ABI 3130 sequencer (Applied Biosystems, Foster City, CA, USA) at Premium Network of Multi-User Equipment/IMT/FMUSP. Chromatograms were analyzed with Sequencher™ 4.7 software (Gene Codes Corporation, Ann Arbor, MI, USA). Genotype assignment utilized Basic Local Alignment Search Tool BLAST (http://blast.ncbi.nlm.nih.gov, accessed on 24 March 2025), Genoma Detective (https://www.genomedetective.com/, accessed on 24 March 2025), Human Calicivirus Typing (HuCaT) (https://calicivirustypingtool.cdc.gov/bctyping.cgi, accessed on 24 March 2025), and Enterovirus Typing Tool Version 0.1 (https://www.rivm.nl/mpf/typingtool/enterovirus, accessed on 24 March 2025).

2.4. Phylogenetic Analysis

The sequences obtained were aligned with prototype sequences of HBoV, NoV, EV, PeV-A, and HAdV retrieved from GenBank using CLUSTAL W in BioEdit Sequence Alignment Editor Software version 7.0.5.2 (Ibis Therapeutics, Carlsbad, CA, USA). Maximum likelihood trees were constructed for each pathogen using MEGA X software [22] with substitution models selected based on the Akaike Information Criterion (AICc). The models used were Tamura-Nei (TN93)+I for HBoV-1, Kimura 2-parameter (K2)+G+I for NoV ORF1, K2+G for NoV ORF2, Hasegawa-Kishino-Yano (HKY)+I for HAdV-C6, K2+G+I for CVA6, and Tamura 3-parameter (T92)+G+I for PeV-A1. Statistical significance for each branching point was assessed with 1000 replicates.

3. Results

3.1. Clinical Findings

Table 1 summarizes clinical findings from 20 patients in the study. The mean and median ages were 1.8 years (range: 11 days to 3 years) and 1 year, respectively. Males accounted for 60% (12/20) of the samples, while females made up 40% (8/20). Diarrhea was the predominant symptom (85%, 17/20), followed by vomiting (60%, 12/20). Fever and coryza were observed in 45% (9/20) and 40% (8/20) of patients, respectively. Less frequently reported symptoms included cough, abdominal pain, productive cough, sore throat, and sneezing. No severe outcomes were reported.

3.2. Viral Diagnosis

Seven different viruses were identified: HBoV, NoV, HAdV, PeV-A, EV, RSV, and Flu A. HBoV and NoV were found in 75% (15/20) of cases, with co-infections observed in 13 patients (65%). These findings suggest their involvement in respiratory illness with gastrointestinal symptoms at SAMEB. Due to limited sample volume, oropharyngeal swabs from three cases (N05, N06 and N07) were excluded from extraction, leaving only fecal samples for analysis. HBoV was detected in both sample types from eight cases, while NoV was exclusively found in stool specimens (Table 1).

HAdV, EV, PeV-A, and RSV were detected in two cases each (10%, 2/20) and Flu A in one case (5%, 1/10). EV was detected in both paired samples (oropharyngeal swab and fecal sample) in positive cases. RSV was found in one case from paired samples and in another case from the swab alone. HAdV and PeV-A were identified exclusively in fecal samples, while Flu A was found only in oropharyngeal swabs. All samples tested negative for RVA, HAstV, and SARS-CoV-2 (Table 1).

Co-infections involving respiratory and enteric viruses were notably high (75%, 15/20). The most common co-infection was HBoV+NoV (40%, 8/20), followed by triple infections including HBoV+NoV+RSV (10%, 2/20), HBoV+NoV+HAdV (10%, 2/20), and others like NoV+PeV-A (5%, 1/20), HBoV+NoV+EV (5%, 1/20), and NoV+EV+PeV-A (5%, 1/20) (Table 1).

3.3. Genotypic Data

Out of 23 HBoV-positive specimens (11 oropharyngeal swabs and 12 fecal samples), 10 (43.5%) were successfully genotyped as HBoV-1. NoV-positive samples exhibited significant genetic diversity; all 15 were classified as genogroup II by RT-qPCR. Sanger sequencing of partial RNA polymerase and capsid regions was successful for 13 samples. The predominant genotype was NoV GII.4_Sydney[P16] (69.2%, 9/13), followed by GII.2[P16] (27.1%, 3/13) and one GII.4_Sydney[P31] strain (7.7%, 1/13). Four sequenced EV samples (two oropharyngeal swabs and two stool samples) were identified as Coxsackievirus A6 (CVA6).

Two fecal HAdV-positive samples were identified as HAdV-C6. Of two PeV-A-positive fecal samples, one was genotyped as PeV-A1 (Table 1).

3.4. Phylogenetic Data

High-quality sequences were selected as representative HBoV strains for phylogenetic analysis. The phylogenetic tree indicated distinct clustering of Brazilian HBoV-1 strains, implying that the HBoV-1 strains associated with respiratory illnesses and gastrointestinal symptoms in children treated at SAMEB do not originate from the same source. Brazilian HBoV-1 sequences showed 99–100% nt among each other. Strain N04/swab grouped with strains from Brazil, Argentina, France, and Japan (2005–2020, 100% nt). Strains N10/swab and N12/swab clustered with those from Brazil, Argentina, Panama, and the Netherlands (2005–2018, 100% nt). Strains N05/swab, N05/feces, and N11/feces clustered with strains from America, Europe, Africa, and Asia (2010–2016, 100% nt) (Figure 1).

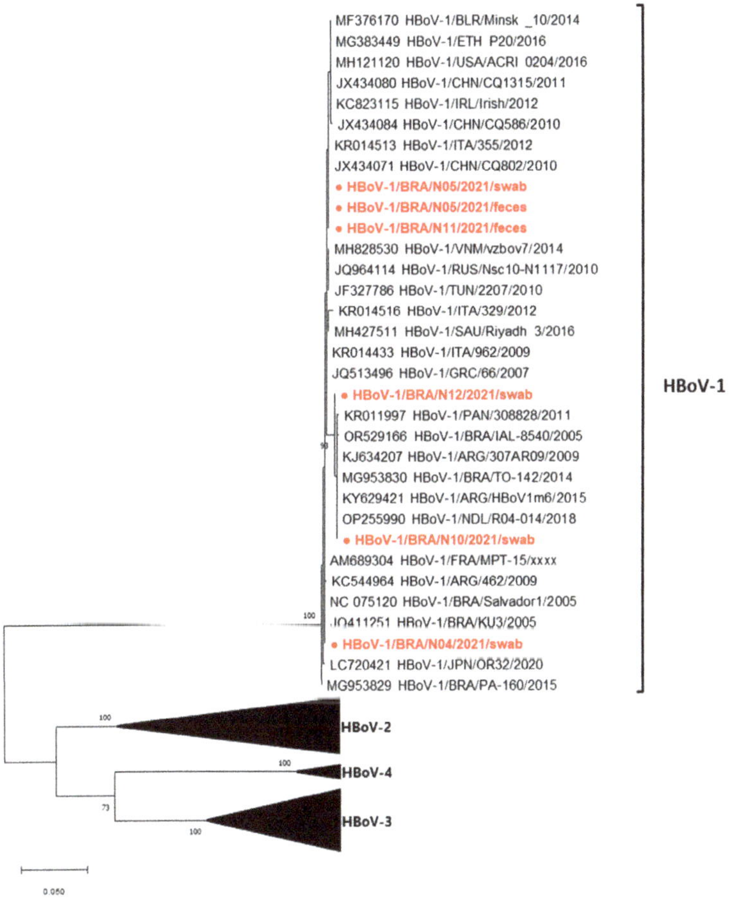

Figure 1. Maximum likelihood phylogenetic tree of the partial VP1/VP2 HBoV-1 protein nucleotide sequence (658-bp fragment) generated with MEGA X software [22] of the Brazilian HBoV-1 strains detected from children with acute respiratory disease and diarrheic symptoms, Barueri, São Paulo, Brazil, 2021 (highlighted in red). HBoV prototype strains were obtained from GenBank database. HBoV assigned genotypes are indicated on the right. Accession numbers of each strain are displayed. The scale indicates the number of divergent nucleotide residues. The percentage of bootstrap values is shown at the branch node.

Phylogenetic trees were constructed using the partial RNA polymerase gene region (282 bp) and capsid region (270 bp) of NoV GII strains. The GII.4_Sydney[P16] ORF2 sequences exhibited 99.1–100% nt and grouped in cluster "c" with other Brazilian sequences from 2021–2022 (Figure 2B). The ORF1 region analysis showed that Brazilian [P16] sequences paired with GII.4 (99.1–100% nt) had a notable affinity with Brazilian strains from 2021–2022 and the Australian strain NSW1705 from 2017 (cluster "a") (Figure 2A). The N04 GII.4_Sydney[P31] strain formed a separate group "b", closely related (99.2–99.4% nt) to Asian and Brazilian sequences from 2017–2021 (Figure 2B). The N04 [P31] ORF1 sequences showed 100% nt with the Brazilian GII.4_Sydney[P31] LVCA31940 strain from 2021 (Figure 2A). Brazilian GII.2[P16] sequences demonstrated 98.4–99.5% nt in ORF1 and 98.5–100% nt in ORF2 with global strains from 2016–2023, and 97.8–100% nt among themselves across both ORFs (Figure 2A,B).

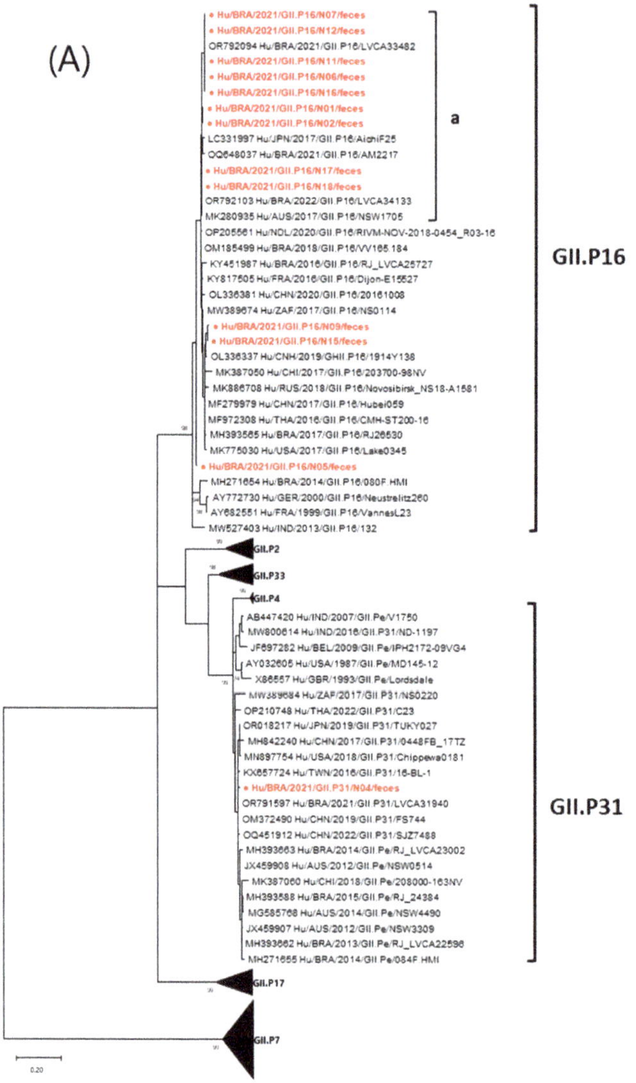

Figure 2. *Cont.*

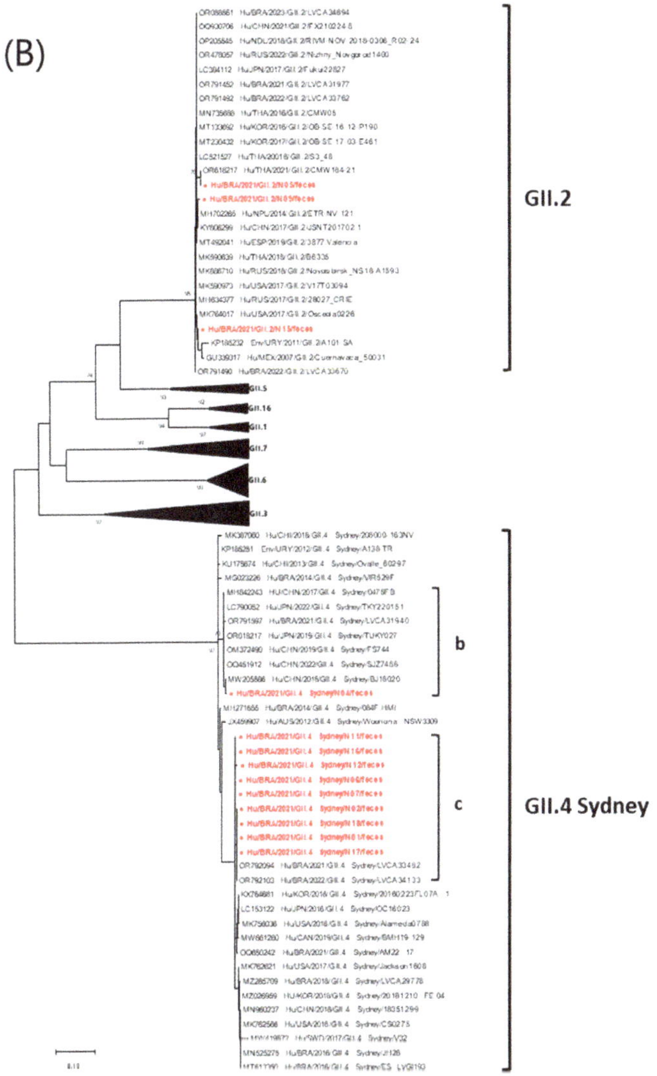

Figure 2. Phylogenetic analysis of Brazilian NoV strains detected from children with acute respiratory disease and diarrheic symptoms, Barueri, São Paulo, Brazil, 2021 (highlighted in red) alongside other selected NoV strains. Maximum-likelihood trees are presented for partial ORF 1 (**A**) and ORF 2 (**B**). Reference NoV sequences were retrieved from the GenBank database, with each strain's accession number, isolate, country, and year indicated. Clusters identified in the present study are denoted by letters a, b, and c. The NoV G-types (ORF2) and P-types (ORF1) are specified. Statistical significance for each branch point was determined using 1000 pseudo-replicate datasets. The scale bar represents nucleotide substitutions per site, and bootstrap values are displayed as percentages at the branch nodes.

The Brazilian HAdV-C6 sequences from N15/feces and N11/swab were closely related, showing 99.8% nt, indicating a common origin. These strains exhibited the highest homology (99.8–100% nt) with the CQHAdV20181126 strain from China, identified in 2018 (Figure 3).

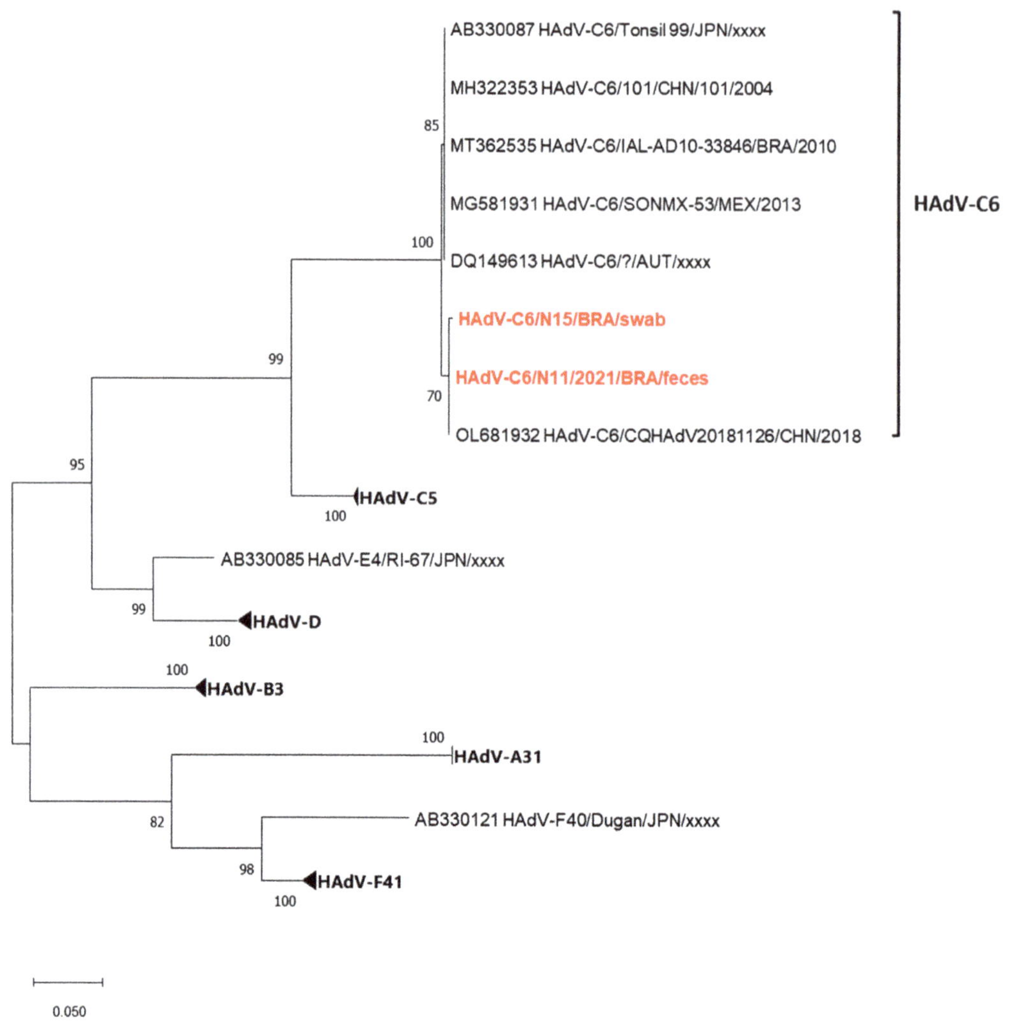

Figure 3. Maximum likelihood phylogenetic tree of the partial Hexon nucleotide (449-bp fragment) generated with MEGA X software [22] of the Brazilian HAdV-C6 strains detected from children with acute respiratory disease and diarrheic symptoms, Barueri, São Paulo, Brazil, 2021 (highlighted in red). HAdV prototype strains were obtained from GenBank database. HAdV assigned genotypes are indicated on the right. Accession numbers of each strain are displayed. The scale indicates the number of divergent nucleotide residues. The percentage of bootstrap values is shown at the branch node.

The Brazilian CVA6 N04 (feces and swab) and N17 (feces and swab) samples were assigned to clade D, sub-lineage D3. The CVA6 lineages (A–D) were classified according to previous proposals [23]. Strains N04/feces and N04/swab (identical sequences) clustered with Brazilian strains from 2019–2021 (98.4–99% nt). Strains N17/feces and N17/swab (identical sequences) grouped with Brazilian strains from 2021 (99.7% nt) and Asian strains from 2017–2019 (95.7–98.1% nt). N04 and N17 strains are remotely related (89.6–89.7% nt), suggesting different origins (Figure 4).

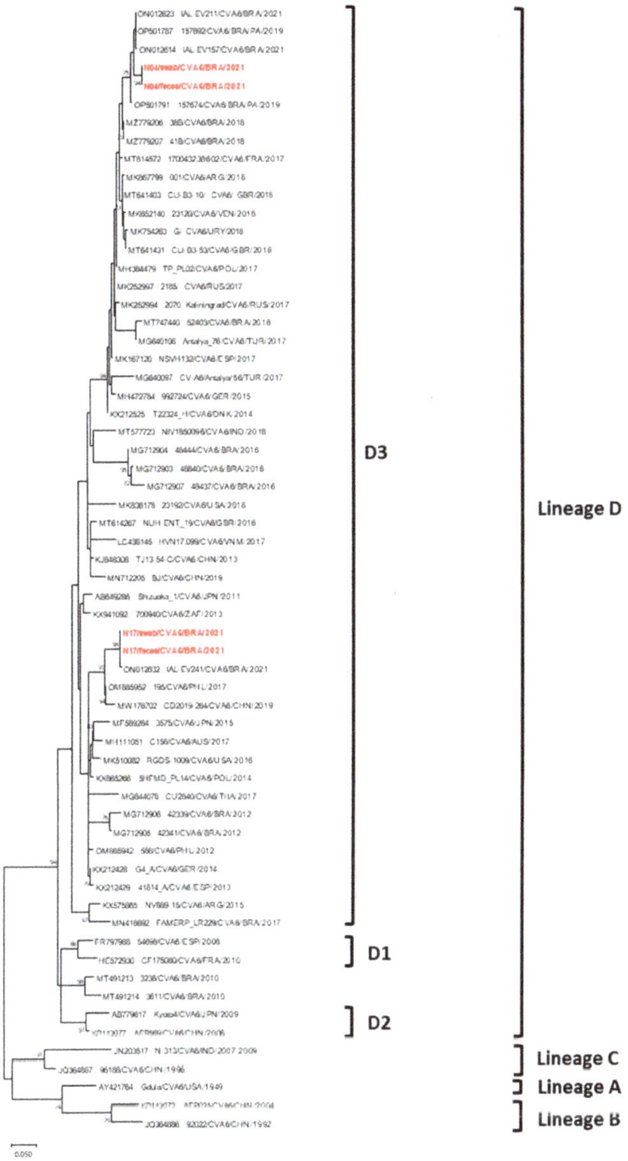

Figure 4. Maximum likelihood phylogenetic tree of the partial VP1 protein nucleotide (334-bp fragment) generated with MEGA X software [22] of the Brazilian CVA6 strains detected from children with acute respiratory disease and diarrheic symptoms, Barueri, São Paulo, Brazil, 2021 (highlighted in red). CVA6 prototype strains were obtained from GenBank database. CVA6 assigned lineages are indicated on the right. Accession numbers of each strain are displayed. The scale indicates the number of divergent nucleotide residues. The percentage of bootstrap values is shown at the branch node.

Phylogenetic analysis of the partial VP1/VP3 junction of a Brazilian PeV-A1 strain shows that the N17/feces/PeV-A1/BRA/2021 strain belongs to subtype HPeV-1B. It is closely related to the Milan_16-227 strain from Italy (2016), with 96.9% nt identity (Figure 5).

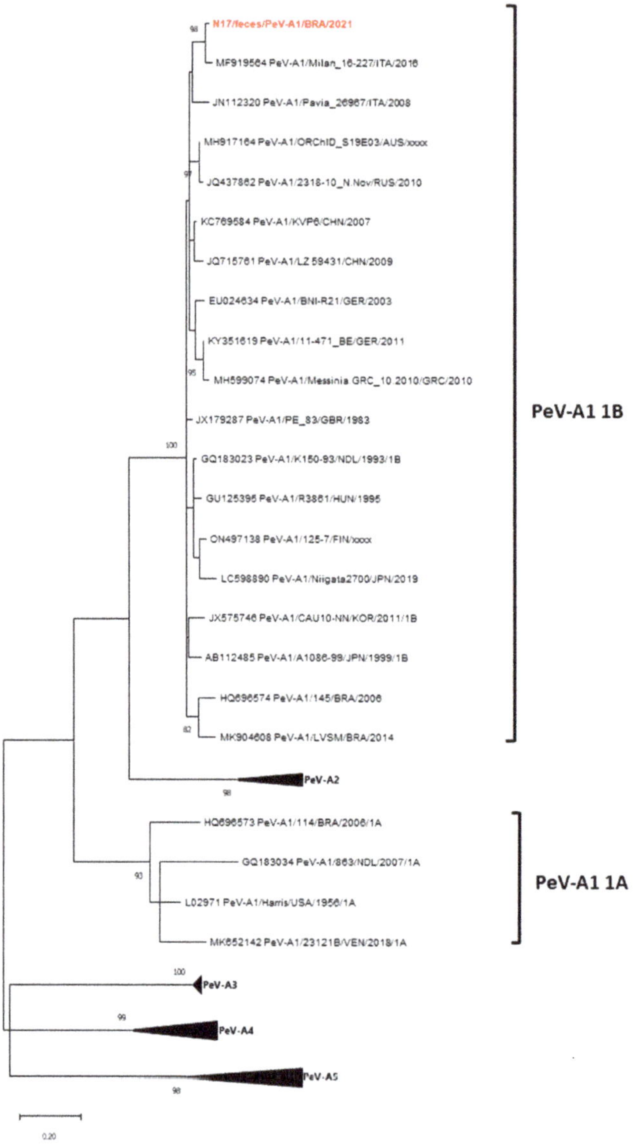

Figure 5. Maximum likelihood phylogenetic tree of the partial VP3/VP1 junction region (280-bp fragment) generated with MEGA X software [22] of the Brazilian PeV-A1 strain detected from children with acute respiratory disease and diarrheic symptoms, Barueri, São Paulo, Brazil, 2021 (highlighted in red). PeV-A prototype strains were obtained from GenBank database. PeV-A1 assigned subtypes are indicated on the right. Accession numbers of each strain are displayed. The scale indicates the number of divergent nucleotide residues. The percentage of bootstrap values is shown at the branch node.

4. Discussion

This study reveals that respiratory illness and gastroenteritis in children in the northwestern metropolitan area of São Paulo during spring 2021 were due to concurrent HBoV (respiratory symptoms) and NoV (gastrointestinal symptoms) infections. Additionally, these children were exposed to other enteric and respiratory pathogens, such as EV, PeV-A, and HAdV. Although mixed viral infections causing gastroenteritis or respiratory illness are globally documented, including in Brazil [24,25], studies on both conditions combined are relatively rare [2,26]. The comprehensive understanding of viral agents responsible for concurrent diarrheal and respiratory illnesses remains notably limited in Brazil. This investigation enhances the understanding of viral agents responsible for concurrent diarrheal and respiratory illnesses in Brazil, offering new perspectives for surveillance efforts.

HBoV infections in patients with influenza-like illness occur year-round, peaking in winter and spring, including in Brazil [6,27], supporting our data. In tropical regions like Brazil, NoV circulates consistently without a seasonal peak [8]. Globally, HBoV often co-infects with other enteric viruses, and studies in Brazil report frequent HBoV and NoV co-circulation [6,28]. However, consensus on the role of HBoV co-infections is difficult due to variations in study designs, inclusion criteria, and the extent of gastroenteric virus testing [28].

HBoV-1 was the only detected genotype, aligning with global findings and underscoring its widespread distribution and strong association with respiratory infections [6,27]. The genetic analysis revealed minimal variability (0.1% nt), consistent with previous studies [29], indicating limited genetic diversity. Despite this low variability, the HBoV-1 strains in this study formed distinct branches, suggesting they do not share a common origin and that there was no ongoing community outbreak of HBoV-1.

Molecular data from NoV strains suggest no outbreak in the studied population but rather an overlap of respiratory and enteric diseases. Three distinct NoV genotypes (GII.4_Sydney[P16], GII.4_Sydney[P31], and GII.2[P16]) were identified, indicating multiple sources of infection. These genotypes are predominant globally and in Brazil [30,31], in agreement with our findings. GII.2[P16] emerged during Japanese outbreaks in 2009–2010, spreading to Asia, Europe, and Australia [32–35], and reaching Brazil in 2017 [8]. GII.4_Sydney[P31] has been prevalent worldwide since 2012, associated with outbreaks, sporadic cases, and asymptomatic infections [36]. The GII.4_Sydney[P16] strain, identified in the US in 2015, also became globally dominant [8,37].

In addition to HBoV and NoV, children in Barueri were co-infected with other fecal and airborne viruses. Despite the presence of mixed infections, the gastroenteritis and respiratory symptoms were mild and similar to those observed in single viral infections. Additionally, it is important to note that the present study involved only an outpatient population treated at a pediatric emergency department, with no severe clinical outcomes or hospitalizations required. The identified HAdV-C6 is a rare type usually linked to respiratory infections [38], with sporadic cases in Brazil [39]. The detection of RSV and Flu A was expected due to the study period aligning with their seasonal occurrence [24].

The study detected two emerging viruses: CVA6 and PeV-A. Since 2008, CVA6 has been linked to a global rise in Hand, Foot, and Mouth Disease (HFMD), including outbreaks in Brazil since 2018 [40,41]. CVA6 has also been associated with central nervous system infections and severe acute respiratory illness [23,42,43]. The two children infected with CVA6 (patients N04 and N17) did not display typical HFMD symptoms, suggesting a link between CVA6 and respiratory symptoms, which is supported by the detection of CVA6 in the swab and feces of both patients, suggesting an ongoing infection. The Brazilian CVA6 strains N04 and N17 identified here exhibit distant genetic relationships. CVA6-N04 strains are genetically linked to those concurrently circulating in Brazil, while CVA6-N17 strains are associated with strains circulating in both Brazil and Asian countries [42,44]. Sub-lineage D3 is the main CVA6 sub-lineage worldwide, associated with HFMD, meningitis, and respiratory diseases [23,41,43].

PeV-A1 was detected in fecal samples from patient N17. PeV-A1 has been associated with both mild respiratory and gastrointestinal infections [45,46], supporting the data obtained here. The original PeV-A1 strain was identified in the USA in 1956 and has since spread globally [7], becoming the most common genotype in many countries [45,46]. Data on PeV-A in Brazil are limited, with little known about the predominant genotypes [47,48]. This study highlights the need for further investigation to understand PeV-A's impact on the health of the Brazilian population, especially children.

No SARS-CoV-2 cases were detected despite the ongoing pandemic. Although COVID-19 vaccination for children under 5 had not begun, isolation measures were eased with daycare centers and schools reopening in Barueri [49], where isolation rates ranged from 28% to 48% during the study (https://www.saopaulo.sp.gov.br/coronavirus/isolamento/, accessed on 28 February 2025). This absence highlights the effectiveness of daycare centers' preventive measures. Reports on HBoV during COVID-19 show varied patterns: some indicate increased rates, others decreased, and some unchanged pre- and post-pandemic [50–52]. Few studies in Brazil have investigated HBoV prevalence during the pandemic [53]. Interestingly, while enveloped viruses like Flu A/B and RSV nearly disappeared, non-enveloped viruses like HBoV, HAdV, and EV were still detected during the pandemic's peak [52], aligning with our findings.

5. Conclusions

Our data indicate that HBoV and NoV caused acute respiratory disease in children $\leq$ 3 years old with diarrhea in northwestern Metropolitan São Paulo in 2021, confirming the overlap between respiratory and enteric diseases. Molecular data suggest no community outbreak, as HBoV and NoV strains showed distinct genotypes and do not share a common origin. The main limitation of this study was the small sample size, resulting from emergency room overcrowding during the COVID-19 outbreak, which led to early discharges and a reduced number of paired sample collections. This constraint impaired a more robust generalization of our findings. Therefore, future studies with larger patient cohorts are warranted to strengthen the validity of our data. Despite the small sample size, multiple viruses were identified, highlighting local viral diversity and high exposure to enteric viruses. Additionally, the cross-sectional design of the present investigation precluded conclusions regarding viral persistence, especially for pathogens like HBoV, which can be shed for prolonged periods [6]. A longitudinal study would be valuable to assess whether the viruses detected represent acute infections or prolonged shedding. These findings underscore the challenges of differential diagnosis due to overlapping symptoms and highlight the importance of syndromic surveillance in capturing the full scope of viral infections in similar clinical settings.

Author Contributions: A.L., N.S.A. and M.L.N. designed the study. L.C.d.R., E.V., L.S.d.A., R.G., Y.F., S.G., A.P., V.C.M.S., A.L.V.d.O., A.H.S.A., B.S.C., N.L.P.F. and A.L.N.d.S. contributed to the study's implementation. NSA collected data and performed clinical evaluations. A.L.V.d.O., A.H.S.A., B.S.C., N.L.P.F. and A.L.N.d.S. were responsible for sample collection, identification, and storage training. L.S.d.A. and R.G. managed sample transportation logistics. A.P. and S.G. standardized Polymerase Chain reactions. A.L. and L.C.d.R. conducted viral screening, while A.L., Y.F. and V.C.M.S. performed sequencing assays. A.L. conducted phylogenetic analysis. N.S.A., L.C.d.R., E.V., L.S.d.A., R.G., Y.F., S.G., A.P., V.C.M.S. and M.L.N. analyzed and interpreted the data. A.L. drafted the manuscript, which was critically revised for intellectual content by N.S.A. and M.L.N. All authors reviewed and approved the final version. A.L. and M.L.N. are the guarantors of the paper. All authors have read and agreed to the published version of the manuscript.

Funding: This study was supported by the Sao Paulo Research Foundation (FAPESP) through grant numbers #2015/12944-9 and #2020/14786-0 to Adriana Luchs, #2021/09064-8 to Yasmin França, and #2022/02529-8 to Ellen Viana. The National Council for Scientific and Technological Development is a government agency under the Ministry of Science and Technology of the Brazilian federal government

(CNPq) #310056/2023-3 to Adriana Luchs. Special Health Fund for Mass Immunization and Disease Control (Fundo Especial de Saúde para Imunização em Massa e Controle de Doenças-FESIMA) CAF N° #001/2021 and #060/2021 to Adriana Luchs. Graduate Support Program—Financial Support for Educational or Research Projects (Programa de Apoio à Pós-Graduação-Auxílio Financeiro a Projeto Educacional ou de Pesquisa-PROAP-AUXPE) #2022/115 to Ellen Viana, Lais Sampaio de Azevedo, and Yasmin França. Coordination for the Improvement of Higher Education Personnel—Scholarship and Support (Management System Coordenação de Aperfeiçoamento de Pessoal de Nível Superior-Sistema de Controle de Bolsas e Auxílio-CAPES-SCBA) #2022-0/88881.689557 to Lais Sampaio de Azevedo. Centers for Research in Emerging Infectious Diseases (CREID) "The Coordinating Research on Emerging Arboviral Threats Encompassing the Neotropics [CREATE-NEO]" 1U01AI151807 to Mauricio Lacerda Nogueira.

Institutional Review Board Statement: Ethics approval was granted by the São José do Rio Preto School of Medicine—FAMERP, São Paulo, Brazil, on 26 February 2024, under protocol number CAAE 81630424.7.0000.5415.

Informed Consent Statement: Informed consent was obtained from all subjects involved in the study.

Data Availability Statement: Nucleotide sequences from this study were submitted to GenBank with accession numbers PP277716-PP277721 (HBoV-1), PP384164-PP384172 (GII.4_Sydney[P16]), PP384190 (GII.4_Sydney[P31]), PP386388-PP386390 (GII.2P[16]), PP429525-PP429526 (HAdV-C6), PP42952-PP429530 (CVA6), and PP496531 (PeV-A1).

Conflicts of Interest: The authors declare no conflicts of interest.

References

1. Bányai, K.; Estes, M.K.; Martella, V.; Parashar, U.D. Viral gastroenteritis. *Lancet* **2018**, *392*, 175–186. [CrossRef]
2. Shen, L.; Yan, H.; Li, W.; Tian, Y.; Lin, C.; Liu, B.; Wang, Y.; Jia, L.; Zhang, D.; Yang, P.; et al. Occurrence of respiratory viruses among outpatients with diarrhea in Beijing, China, 2019–2020. *Front. Microbiol.* **2023**, *13*, 1073980. [CrossRef]
3. Wang, J.; Li, F.; Wei, H.; Lian, Z.X.; Sun, R.; Tian, Z. Respiratory influenza virus infection induces intestinal immune injury via microbiota-mediated Th17 cell-dependent inflammation. *J. Exp. Med.* **2014**, *211*, 2397–2410. [CrossRef]
4. Rao, C.D. Enteroviruses in gastrointestinal diseases. *Rev. Med. Virol.* **2021**, *31*, 1–12. [CrossRef]
5. Pérez-Martínez, Z.; Álvarez-Argüelles, M.E.; Rojo-Alba, S.; Castello-Abietar, C.; Boga, J.A.; Morilla-Morilla, A.; Vivanco-Allende, A.; Rodríguez-Suárez, J.; Alonso-Álvarez, M.A.; Melón, S. Incidence of enterovirus in patients with acute gastroenteritis. *Eur. J. Clin. Microbiol. Infect. Dis.* **2021**, *40*, 2185–2190. [CrossRef] [PubMed]
6. Guido, M.; Tumolo, M.R.; Verri, T.; Romano, A.; Serio, F.; De Giorgi, M.; De Donno, A.; Bagordo, F.; Zizza, A. Human bocavirus: Current knowledge and future challenges. *World J. Gastroenterol.* **2016**, *22*, 8684–8697. [CrossRef] [PubMed]
7. de Crom, S.C.; Rossen, J.W.; van Furth, A.M.; Obihara, C.C. Enterovirus and parechovirus infection in children: A brief overview. *Eur. J. Pediatr.* **2016**, *175*, 1023–1029. [CrossRef]
8. Sarmento, S.K.; de Andrade, J.D.S.R.; Miagostovich, M.P.; Fumian, T.M. Virological and Epidemiological Features of Norovirus Infections in Brazil, 2017–2018. *Viruses* **2021**, *13*, 1724. [CrossRef]
9. Silva, A.D.D.; Veiga, A.B.G.D.; Cruz, O.G.; Bastos, L.S.; Gomes, M.F.D.C. Severe acute respiratory infection surveillance in Brazil: The role of public, private and philanthropic healthcare units. *Health Policy Plan.* **2022**, *37*, 1075–1085. [CrossRef]
10. Zeng, S.Q.; Halkosalo, A.; Salminen, M.; Szakal, E.D.; Puustinen, L.; Vesikari, T. One-step quantitative RT-PCR for the detection of rotavirus in acute gastroenteritis. *J. Virol. Methods* **2008**, *153*, 238–240. [CrossRef]
11. Zhang, S.; Wang, J.; Yan, Q.; He, S.; Zhou, W.; Ge, S.; Xia, N. A one-step, triplex, real-time RT-PCR assay for the simultaneous detection of enterovirus 71, coxsackie A16 and pan-enterovirus in a single tube. *PLoS ONE.* **2014**, *9*, e102724. [CrossRef]
12. Kageyama, T.; Kojima, S.; Shinohara, M.; Uchida, K.; Fukushi, S.; Hoshino, F.B.; Takeda, N.; Katayama, K. Broadly reactive and highly sensitive assay for Norwalk-like viruses based on real-time quantitative reverse transcription-PCR. *J. Clin. Microbiol.* **2003**, *41*, 1548–1557. [CrossRef] [PubMed]
13. Nix, W.A.; Maher, K.; Johansson, E.S.; Niklasson, B.; Lindberg, A.M.; Pallansch, M.A.; Oberste, M.S. Detection of all known parechoviruses by real-time PCR. *J. Clin. Microbiol.* **2008**, *46*, 2519–2524. [CrossRef]
14. Heim, A.; Ebnet, C.; Harste, G.; Pring-Akerblom, P. Rapid and quantitative detection of human adenovirus DNA by real-time PCR. *J. Med. Virol.* **2003**, *70*, 228–239. [CrossRef] [PubMed]
15. Lu, X.; Chittaganpitch, M.; Olsen, S.J.; Mackay, I.M.; Sloots, T.P.; Fry, A.M.; Erdman, D.D. Real-time PCR assays for detection of bocavirus in human specimens. *J. Clin. Microbiol.* **2006**, *44*, 3231–3235. [CrossRef]

16. Chu, D.K.; Poon, L.L.; Guan, Y.; Peiris, J.S. Novel astroviruses in insectivorous bats. *J. Virol.* **2008**, *82*, 9107–9114. [CrossRef] [PubMed]
17. Xu, W.; McDonough, M.C.; Erdman, D.D. Species-specific identification of human adenoviruses by a multiplex PCR assay. *J. Clin. Microbiol.* **2000**, *38*, 4114–4120. [CrossRef]
18. Durigon, G.S.; Oliveira, D.B.; Vollet, S.B.; Storni, J.G.; Felício, M.C.; Finelli, C.; Piera, J.; Magalhães, M.; Caldeira, R.N.; Barbosa, M.L.; et al. Hospital-acquired human bocavirus in infants. *J. Hosp. Infect.* **2010**, *76*, 171–173. [CrossRef]
19. Chhabra, P.; Browne, H.; Huynh, T.; Diez-Valcarce, M.; Barclay, L.; Kosek, M.N.; Ahmed, T.; Lopez, M.R.; Pan, C.Y.; Vinjé, J. Single-step RT-PCR assay for dual genotyping of GI and GII norovirus strains. *J. Clin. Virol.* **2021**, *134*, 104689. [CrossRef]
20. Iturriza-Gómara, M.; Megson, B.; Gray, J. Molecular detection and characterization of human enteroviruses directly from clinical samples using RT-PCR and DNA sequencing. *J. Med. Virol.* **2006**, *78*, 243–253. [CrossRef]
21. Ghanem-Zoubi, N.; Shiner, M.; Shulman, L.M.; Sofer, D.; Wolf, D.; Marva, E.; Kra-Oz, Z.; Shachor-Meyouhas, Y.; Averbuch, D.; Bechor-Fellner, A.; et al. Human parechovirus type 3 central nervous system infections in Israeli infants. *J. Clin. Virol.* **2013**, *58*, 205–210. [CrossRef] [PubMed]
22. Kumar, S.; Stecher, G.; Li, M.; Knyaz, C.; Tamura, K. MEGA X: Molecular Evolutionary Genetics Analysis across Computing Platforms. *Mol. Biol. Evol.* **2018**, *35*, 1547–1549. [CrossRef]
23. Hellferscee, O.; Tempia, S.; Walaza, S.; Variava, E.; Dawood, H.; Wolter, N.; Madhi, S.A.; du Plessis, M.; Cohen, C.; Treurnicht, F.K. Enterovirus genotypes among patients with severe acute respiratory illness, influenza-like illness, and asymptomatic individuals in South Africa, 2012–2014. *J. Med. Virol.* **2017**, *89*, 1759–1767. [CrossRef] [PubMed]
24. Albuquerque, M.C.; Varella, R.B.; Santos, N. Acute respiratory viral infections in children in Rio de Janeiro and Teresópolis, Brazil. *Rev. Inst. Med. Trop. Sao Paulo* **2012**, *54*, 249–255. [CrossRef] [PubMed]
25. Swets, M.C.; Russell, C.D.; Harrison, E.M.; Docherty, A.B.; Lone, N.; Girvan, M.; Hardwick, H.E.; ISARIC4C Investigators; Visser, L.G.; Openshaw, P.J.M.; et al. SARS-CoV-2 co-infection with influenza viruses, respiratory syncytial virus, or adenoviruses. *Lancet* **2022**, *399*, 1463–1464. [CrossRef]
26. Velasco, J.M.; Yoon, I.K.; Mason, C.J.; Jarman, R.G.; Bodhidatta, L.; Klungthong, C.; Silapong, S.; Valderama, M.T.; Wongstitwilairoong, T.; Torres, A.G.; et al. Applications of PCR (real-time and MassTag) and enzyme-linked immunosorbent assay in diagnosis of respiratory infections and diarrheal illness among deployed U.S. military personnel during exercise Balikatan 2009, Philippines. *Mil. Med.* **2011**, *176*, 1096–1100. [CrossRef]
27. Silva, P.E.; Figueiredo, C.A.; Luchs, A.; de Paiva, T.M.; Pinho, M.A.B.; Paulino, R.S.; da Silva, D.B.B.; de Oliveira Santos, K.C.; Afonso, A.M.S.; de Oliveira, M.I. Human bocavirus in hospitalized children under 5 years with acute respiratory infection, São Paulo, Brazil, 2010. *Arch. Virol.* **2018**, *163*, 1325–1330. [CrossRef]
28. Viana, E.; França, Y.; de Azevedo, L.S.; Medeiros, R.S.; Guiducci, R.; Guadagnucci, S.; Luchs, A. Genotypic diversity and long-term impact of human bocavirus on diarrheal disease: Insights from historical fecal samples in Brazil. *J. Med. Virol.* **2024**, *96*, e29429. [CrossRef]
29. Kapoor, A.; Simmonds, P.; Slikas, E.; Li, L.; Bodhidatta, L.; Sethabutr, O.; Triki, H.; Bahri, O.; Oderinde, B.S.; Baba, M.M.; et al. Human bocaviruses are highly diverse, dispersed, recombination prone, and prevalent in enteric infections. *J. Infect. Dis.* **2010**, *201*, 1633–1643. [CrossRef]
30. Zheng, G.L.; Zhu, Z.X.; Cui, J.L.; Yu, J.M. Evolutionary analyses of emerging GII.2[P16] and GII.4 Sydney [P16] noroviruses. *Virus Evol.* **2022**, *8*, veac030. [CrossRef]
31. Sarmento, S.K.; de Andrade, J.D.S.R.; Malta, F.C.; Fialho, A.M.; Mello, M.S.; Burlandy, F.M.; Fumian, T.M. Norovirus Epidemiology and Genotype Circulation during the COVID-19 Pandemic in Brazil, 2019–2022. *Pathogens* **2023**, *13*, 3. [CrossRef] [PubMed]
32. Iritani, N.; Kaida, A.; Abe, N.; Sekiguchi, J.; Kubo, H.; Takakura, K.; Goto, K.; Ogura, H.; Seto, Y. Increase of GII.2 norovirus infections during the 2009-2010 season in Osaka City, Japan. *J. Med. Virol.* **2012**, *84*, 517–525. [CrossRef]
33. Jin, M.; Wu, S.; Kong, X.; Xie, H.; Fu, J.; He, Y.; Feng, W.; Liu, N.; Li, J.; Rainey, J.J.; et al. Norovirus Outbreak Surveillance, China, 2016–2018. *Emerg. Infect. Dis.* **2020**, *26*, 437–445. [CrossRef] [PubMed]
34. Bidalot, M.; Théry, L.; Kaplon, J.; De Rougemont, A.; Ambert-Balay, K. Emergence of new recombinant noroviruses GII.p16-GII.4 and GII.p16-GII.2, France, winter 2016 to 2017. *Euro Surveill.* **2017**, *22*, 30508. [CrossRef] [PubMed]
35. Bruggink, L.D.; Triantafilou, M.J.; Marshall, J.A. The molecular epidemiology of norovirus outbreaks in Victoria, 2016. *Commun Dis Intell.* **2018**, *42*, s2209–s6051.
36. Van Beek, J.; de Graaf, M.; Al-Hello, H.; Allen, D.J.; Ambert-Balay, K.; Botteldoorn, N.; Brytting, M.; Buesa, J.; Cabrerizo, M.; Chan, M.; et al. Molecular surveillance of norovirus, 2005–16: An epidemiological analysis of data collected from the NoroNet network. *Lancet Infect. Dis.* **2018**, *18*, 545–553. [CrossRef]
37. Cannon, J.L.; Bonifacio, J.; Bucardo, F.; Buesa, J.; Bruggink, L.; Chan, M.C.; Fumian, T.M.; Giri, S.; Gonzalez, M.D.; Hewitt, J.; et al. Global Trends in Norovirus Genotype Distribution among Children with Acute Gastroenteritis. *Emerg. Infect. Dis.* **2021**, *27*, 1438–1445. [CrossRef]

38. Shen, C.F.; Wang, S.M.; Wang, J.R.; Hu, Y.S.; Ho, T.S.; Liu, C.C. Comparative study of clinical and epidemiological characteristics of major pediatric adenovirus epidemics in southern Taiwan. *BMC Infect. Dis.* **2019**, *19*, 681. [CrossRef]
39. Souza, E.V.; de Souza, Y.F.V.P.; Medeiros, R.S.; de Azevedo, L.S.; de Queiroz, T.G.A.; Sanz-Duro, R.L.; Marinho, R.D.S.S.; Komninakis, S.V.; Timenetsky, M.D.C.S.T.; Luchs, A. Diversity of enteric and non-enteric human adenovirus strains in Brazil, 2006–2011. *Arch. Virol.* **2021**, *166*, 897–903. [CrossRef]
40. Kimmis, B.D.; Downing, C.; Tyring, S. Hand-foot-and-mouth disease caused by coxsackievirus A6 on the rise. *Cutis* **2018**, *102*, 353–356.
41. Luchs, A.; Azevedo, L.S.; Souza, E.V.; Medeiros, R.S.; Souza, Y.F.V.P.; Teixeira, D.L.F.; Carneiro, T.F.O.; Alencar, G.M.F.; Morais, F.L.S.L.; Pinto, D.F.A.; et al. Coxsackievirus A6 strains causing an outbreak of hand-foot-and-mouth disease in Northeastern Brazil in 2018. *Rev. Inst. Med. Trop. Sao Paulo* **2022**, *64*, e16. [CrossRef]
42. Justino, M.C.A.; Mesquita, D.S.; Souza, M.F.; Farias, F.P.; Alves, J.C.D.S.; Ferreira, J.L.; Lopes, D.P.; Tavares, F.N. Atypical hand-foot-mouth disease in Belém, Amazon region, northern Brazil, with detection of coxsackievirus A6. *J. Clin. Virol.* **2020**, *126*, 104307. [CrossRef] [PubMed]
43. Rocha, L.C.D.; Estofolete, C.F.; Milhim, B.H.G.A.; Augusto, M.T.; Zini, N.; Silva, G.C.D.D.; Ferraz-Junior, H.C.; Brienze, V.M.S.; Liso, E.; Cunha, M.S.; et al. Enteric viruses circulating in undiagnosed central nervous system infections at tertiary hospital in São José do Rio Preto, São Paulo, Brazil. *J. Med. Virol.* **2021**, *93*, 3539–3548. [CrossRef]
44. Foronda, J.L.M.; Jiao, M.M.A.D.; Climacosa, F.M.M.; Oshitani, H.; Apostol, L.N.G. Epidemiological and molecular characterization of Coxsackievirus A6 causing hand, foot, and mouth disease in the Philippines, 2012–2017. *Infect. Genet. Evol.* **2023**, *114*, 105498. [CrossRef]
45. Malasao, R.; Khamrin, P.; Kumthip, K.; Ushijima, H.; Maneekarn, N. Molecular epidemiology and genetic diversity of human parechoviruses in children hospitalized with acute diarrhea in Thailand during 2011–2016. *Arch. Virol.* **2019**, *164*, 1743–1752. [CrossRef] [PubMed]
46. Skanke, L.H.; Lysvand, H.; Heimdal, I.; Moe, N.; Krokstad, S.; Christensen, A.; Risnes, K.; Nordbø, S.A.; Døllner, H. Parechovirus A in Hospitalized Children with Respiratory Tract Infections: A 10-Year-Long Study from Norway. *J. Pediatric Infect. Dis. Soc.* **2021**, *10*, 722–729. [CrossRef] [PubMed]
47. Drexler, J.F.; Grywna, K.; Stöcker, A.; Almeida, P.S.; Medrado-Ribeiro, T.C.; Eschbach-Bludau, M.; Petersen, N.; da Costa-Ribeiro, H.J.; Drosten, C. Novel human parechovirus from Brazil. *Emerg. Infect. Dis.* **2009**, *15*, 310–313. [CrossRef]
48. Leal, É.; Luchs, A.; Milagres, F.A.P.; Komninakis, S.V.; Gill, D.E.; Lobato, M.C.A.B.S.; Brustulin, R.; Chagas, R.T.D.; Abrão, M.F.N.D.S.; Soares, C.V.D.A.; et al. Recombinant Strains of Human Parechovirus in Rural Areas in the North of Brazil. *Viruses* **2019**, *11*, 488. [CrossRef]
49. Soares, G.D.S.; Morais, L.V.; Silva, K.C.N.; Ferreira, E.M.; Shio, M.T.; Romano, C.M.; Conde, C.R.; Sabino, E.C.; França, C.N.; Nali, L.H. Low frequency of SARS-CoV2 infection in daycare centers during the reopening of school activities in the Southeast's poor area of Brazil. *Rev. Inst. Med. Trop. São Paulo* **2022**, *64*, e46. [CrossRef]
50. Yum, S.; Hong, K.; Sohn, S.; Kim, J.; Chun, B.C. Trends in Viral Respiratory Infections During COVID-19 Pandemic, South Korea. *Emerg. Infect. Dis.* **2021**, *27*, 1685–1688. [CrossRef]
51. Ippolito, G.; La Vecchia, A.; Umbrello, G.; Di Pietro, G.; Bono, P.; Scalia Catenacci, S.; Pinzani, R.; Tagliabue, C.; Bosis, S.; Agostoni, C.; et al. Disappearance of Seasonal Respiratory Viruses in Children Under Two Years Old During COVID-19 Pandemic: A Monocentric Retrospective Study in Milan, Italy. *Front. Pediatr.* **2021**, *9*, 721005. [CrossRef] [PubMed]
52. Cho, H.J.; Rhee, J.E.; Kang, D.; Choi, E.H.; Lee, N.J.; Woo, S.; Lee, J.; Lee, S.-W.; Kim, E.-J., Yun, K.W. Epidemiology of Respiratory Viruses in Korean Children Before and After the COVID-19 Pandemic: A Prospective Study from National Surveillance System. *J. Korean Med. Sci.* **2024**, *39*, e171. [CrossRef] [PubMed]
53. Fontes, V.; Ferreira, H.; Ribeiro, M.; Pinheiro, A.; Maramaldo, C.; Pereira, E.; Batista, L.; Júnior, A.; Lobato, L.; Silva, F.; et al. High Incidence of Respiratory Syncytial Virus in Children with Community-Acquired Pneumonia from a City in the Brazilian Pre-Amazon Region. *Viruses* **2023**, *15*, 1306. [CrossRef] [PubMed]

viruses

MDPI

Article

Trends in Norovirus Genotypes in South Korea, 2019–2024: Insights from Nationwide Dual Typing Surveillance

Minji Lee, Seung-Rye Cho, Yunhee Jo, Deog-Yong Lee, Myung-Guk Han and Sun-Whan Park *

Division of Viral Diseases, Department of Diagnosis and Analysis, Korea Disease Control and Prevention Agency, Cheongju 28159, Republic of Korea

* Correspondence: sunwhan@korea.kr; Tel.: +82-43-719-8193

Abstract

Noroviruses are a leading cause of acute gastroenteritis worldwide, with a particularly high burden among children under five years of age. We analyzed nationwide surveillance data from EnterNet-Korea collected between 2019 and 2024—covering both the pre- and post-COVID-19 pandemic periods—to assess norovirus detection rates and genotype distribution. Noroviruses were detected by RT-qPCR, and dual genotyping of capsid (G) and polymerase (P) types was performed by sequencing the ORF1–2 junction region. Among the 67,159 specimens tested, 8.4% (n = 5652) were norovirus-positive, with the highest prevalence observed in children aged 0–5 years (19.9%). In this age group, genotyping was successful in 72.4% (2633/3635) of positive cases, identifying 30 distinct genotypes (GI: 9; GII: 21). The most common strains were GII.4[P31] (38.1%), GII.4[P16] (27.1%), and GII.2[P16] (10.4%), with substantial year-to-year variation. Notably, the emergence of GII.17[P17] in late 2024 indicates shifting genotype dynamics, underscoring the need for strengthened surveillance and reconsideration of vaccine strain selection. To our knowledge, this is the first nationwide dual-typing study in Korea encompassing the COVID-19 pandemic era. These findings provide essential baseline data for integration into global surveillance systems and inform future vaccine development and public health strategies.

Keywords: norovirus; acute gastroenteritis; molecular epidemiology; RdRp–VP1 junction; surveillance

1. Introduction

Noroviruses are recognized as one of the leading causes of acute gastroenteritis across all age groups worldwide, with a particularly high incidence among children under five years of age [1–4]. Owing to their low infective dose and multiple routes of transmission, they can spread rapidly and cause outbreaks in community and healthcare settings [1,5,6]. Noroviruses are non-enveloped, single-stranded RNA viruses belonging to the family *Caliciviridae*, with a positive-sense RNA genome of approximately 7.5 kb in length [1]. The genome consists of three open reading frames (ORFs): ORF1 encodes the nonstructural proteins, ORF2 encodes the major capsid protein VP1, and ORF3 encodes the minor structural protein VP2 [1,7,8].

Currently, the noroviruses identified are classified into ten genogroups (GI–GX), among which GI, GII, GIV, GVIII, and GIX are known to infect humans [1,9]. Each genogroup is further subdivided into capsid genotypes (G types), based on the major capsid protein (VP1) gene, and polymerase genotypes (P types), based on the RNA-dependent RNA polymerase (RdRp) gene in the ORF1 region [10]. In 2019, Chhabra et al. proposed a revised classification system using globally accumulated norovirus sequence data [10]. Based on this classification, nine capsid genotypes have been identified within GI, and more than 27 have been identified within GII, while 14 P types in GI and more than 37 in GII have been reported. GII.4 has been the most predominant genotype over the past several decades, continually generating novel variants through recombination with diverse RdRp types [11]. Such recombination events are associated with antigenic variation and enhanced epidemic potential [10,12]. Consequently, the dual typing system, which designates both VP1-based genotypes and RdRp-based P types, has been adopted as the standard classification approach for elucidating the molecular epidemiology and evolutionary dynamics of noroviruses [10,13].

Molecular epidemiological surveillance of noroviruses has been systematically implemented worldwide through national and regional networks. In the United States, CaliciNet serves as the primary surveillance platform, enabling real-time collection and analysis of sequence data from norovirus cases to monitor the emergence of epidemic genotypes and recombination events [14,15]. In Europe and other regions, NoroNet is a collaborative network involving multiple public health institutes and research laboratories, facilitating comprehensive monitoring of genotype distribution and epidemic trends [16]. In the Asia-Pacific region, the NoroNet Asia-Pacific branch provides region-specific epidemiological insights through cross-border data sharing [17,18]. Collectively, these international surveillance systems play a pivotal role in the timely detection of novel variants, the formulation of response strategies, and the establishment of baseline data essential for vaccine development. In Korea, the Korea Disease Control and Prevention Agency (KDCA) operates the "Enteric pathogen surveillance Network (EnterNet-Korea)" laboratory-based surveillance system in collaboration with primary and secondary healthcare facilities, which systematically monitors the incidence of acute diarrheal diseases and the distribution of their causative agents. This program encompasses comprehensive analyses of detection trends for noroviruses, alongside 10 bacterial genera, 5 viral pathogens, and 4 protozoa associated with acute gastroenteritis.

During the COVID-19 pandemic, the widespread implementation of non-pharmaceutical interventions (NPIs), including social distancing, mask-wearing, and enhanced hand hygiene, influenced not only the transmission of respiratory viruses but also the circulation of enteric viruses such as norovirus [7,19–22]. In Korea, similar reductions were also observed for other enteric viruses such as rotavirus and adenovirus during the pandemic, supporting the notion that NPIs substantially altered the epidemiology of multiple AGE-associated pathogens.

Previous molecular epidemiological studies conducted in Korea have primarily relied on partial capsid genotyping and were often limited to short study periods or regional data. Comprehensive nationwide surveillance applying dual typing and capturing the effects of the COVID-19 pandemic has not been reported.

This study quantitatively analyzed nationwide sentinel surveillance data to assess temporal changes in norovirus detection rates and genotype distribution over a six-year period between January 2019 and December 2024, encompassing the unique public health context of the COVID-19 pandemic. Notably, unlike previous studies in Korea that primarily focused on capsid genotyping, this is the first nationwide investigation to apply dual typing, thereby providing significant academic value and critical baseline information for future vaccine development and surveillance strategies. In addition, given rapid shifts in genotype predominance and the emergence of novel variants, continuous nationwide monitoring is essential not only for academic purposes but also for guiding vaccine strain selection and strengthening preparedness against foodborne and waterborne outbreaks in Korea.

2. Materials & Methods

2.1. Stool Sample Collection

Fecal or rectal swab specimens were collected from outpatients presenting with acute gastroenteritis (AGE) symptoms between January 2019 and December 2024. AGE was defined as the occurrence of three or more episodes of watery diarrhea per day, vomiting, nausea, and/or fever (≥37.8 °C, measured orally), which are the major clinical features of water- and foodborne infectious diseases. Specimens were obtained from patients at 76 hospitals participating in EnterNet-Korea. During the study period, minor changes occurred in the number of participating medical institutions (≤10), and the Sejong Institute of Health and Environment joined this study in August 2022. Nevertheless, the specimen collection system and diagnostic protocols remained consistent throughout the study period. Laboratory testing was performed at 18 provincial and metropolitan Institutes of Health and Environment according to the national standard operating procedures. Each institute regularly participated in external quality assessments organized by the Korea Disease Control and Prevention Agency (KDCA) to ensure testing proficiency and reliability of results. All specimens were collected as part of routine national public health surveillance conducted by the KDCA. No identifiable patient information was included in the data. In accordance with institutional policy, analyses conducted for public health surveillance are not considered human-subject research; therefore, institutional review board approval and informed consent were not required for this study.

2.2. Norovirus Detection

For fecal specimens, 1 g stool sample was suspended in 9 mL of 0.1 M phosphate-buffered saline (PBS), while 3 mL of PBS was added to rectal swab specimens. The suspensions were vortexed for 3 min to ensure thorough homogenization. Each fecal suspension was centrifuged at 12,000 rpm for 10 min at 4 °C, and the supernatant was collected for nucleic acid extraction. Viral nucleic acids were extracted using the NucleoMag Viral RNA/DNA Isolation Kit (Macherey-Nagel, Düren, 52355, Germany) according to the manufacturer's instructions. Noroviruses were detected quantitative real-time reverse transcription PCR (qRT-PCR) based on the national standard method. qRT-PCR detection was performed with a commercial TaqMan assay (PowerChek™ Norovirus GI/GII Multiplex Real-Time PCR Kit, Kogene, Korea; cat. no. IR1200F) on an ABI 7500 Real-Time PCR System. Cycling: 50 °C 30 min (reverse transcription), 95 °C 10 min, then 45 cycles of 95 °C 15 s and 55 °C 60 s. Per laboratory SOP, positivity thresholds were Ct ≤ 37.2 (GI) and Ct ≤ 37.7 (GII). Specimens with Ct ≥ 36 were repeat-tested; concordant results were retained and discordant results classified as negative.

Genotyping targeted the RdRp–VP1 junction using established primers (GI: Mon432/G1SKR; GII: Mon431/G2SKR) with Sanger sequencing. Nucleotide sequences obtained in this study were submitted to NCBI GenBank (accession numbers: PX598973-PX598992, PX599239-PX599306, PX599383-PX599529, PX599585-PX599634, PX599732-PX599767, PX599773-PX599997).

2.3. Norovirus Genotyping

Genotyping was performed on specimens that tested positive for norovirus by qRT-PCR. For samples collected between January 2022 and December 2024, dual typing of the RNA-dependent RNA polymerase (RdRp) and capsid junction region was carried out immediately after qRT-PCR, using previously reported primer sets (GI: Mon432/G1SKR; GII: Mon431/G2SKR) [23]. For samples collected between 2019 and December 2021, only the capsid region had been analyzed at the time of detection; therefore, polymerase typing was retrospectively performed. PCR products were subjected to Sanger sequencing by a commercial sequencing service provider, and nucleotide sequences were obtained. The sequences were aligned and edited using the MEGA software package. Norovirus genotypes were determined according to the updated nomenclature system using two publicly available tools: the Calicivirus Typing Tool (https://calicivirustypingtool.cdc.gov/, accessed 30 June 2025) and the Norovirus Typing Tool provided by RIVM (https://mpf.rivm.nl/mpf/typingtool/norovirus, accessed on 30 June 2025). Sequences with insufficient reading quality or ambiguous base calls were excluded from analysis. Potential recombinant strains were screened using the RIVM Norovirus Typing Tool and confirmed by phylogenetic analysis of the partial RdRp and VP1 regions.

2.4. Statistical Analysis

The norovirus detection rate was calculated as the proportion of positive samples relative to the total number of specimens tested each year. Age-specific analyses were stratified into four groups (0–5 years, 6–15 years, 16–59 years, and ≥60 years), and the detection rate was determined based on the total number of samples tested within each group. For regional analysis, specimens were categorized according to the hospitals and laboratories participating in surveillance, and detection rates were calculated as the number of positive samples relative to the total tested within each region. Genotype analysis was performed on norovirus-positive samples from the 0–5 year age group. Samples lacking key patient information (e.g., age or collection date) were excluded from statistical analyses. To assess whether detection rates differed significantly across categories, a chi-square test for proportions was conducted using R (R Foundation for Statistical Computing, Vienna, Austria) and Python 3.11.5 (Python Software Foundation, Wilmington, DE, USA). A p-value of <0.05 was considered statistically significant for all analyses. Temporal trends in annual detection rates were assessed using the Cochran–Armitage trend test. All statistical analyses were performed with a significance threshold of $p < 0.05$.

3. Results

3.1. Norovirus Detection Rate

Norovirus was detected in 8.4% (n = 5652) of the samples. Among the positive cases, genogroup II (GII) accounted for 93.3% (5271/5652), while genogroup I (GI) was detected in 9.0% (n = 509). GI and GII were co-detected in 2.3% (n = 128) of the samples. Age-specific analysis revealed highest detection rate in the 0–5-year age group, with 19.9% (3635/18,291) positivity, representing 64.3% (3635/5652) of all positive cases (Table 1). Detection rates decreased progressively with increasing age. Although the ≥60 year age group contributed the largest number of tested samples (26,755/67,159), it exhibited the lowest positivity rate at 1.7% (443/26,755). Regionally, the highest norovirus detection rates were observed in Gwangju (24.4%), Seoul (15.7%), and Daejeon (10.6%), whereas the lowest rates were reported in Chungbuk (2.1%), Gyeongnam (2.8%), and Jeju (2.8%). Detailed regional detection data are provided in Supplementary Table S1. In particular, southwestern provinces such as Gwangju consistently showed the highest detection rates across all years, whereas provinces including Chungbuk, Gyeongnam, and Jeju maintained rates below 3%, suggesting potential geographic heterogeneity in norovirus transmission dynamics. Although genotype analysis focused on the 0–5 year age group, preliminary sequencing of a subset of older patients indicated similar predominance of GII.4 variants but with reduced genotype diversity, suggesting possible age-related differences in strain circulation.

Table 1. Age-wise norovirus detection rate among acute gastroenteritis cases in South Korea during 2019–2024. Data are presented as the number of positive samples over the total tested, with percentages in parentheses.

Age	No. of Samples—NoV Positive/Tested (%)						
	2019	2020	2021	2022	2023	2024	Total
0–5	530/2798 (18.9)	324/2258 (14.3)	637/3262 (19.5)	803/3463 (23.2)	721/3633 (19.8)	620/2877 (21.6)	3635/18,291 (19.9)
6–15	98/951 (10.3)	74/874 (8.5)	169/1090 (15.5)	116/1083 (10.7)	149/1398 (10.7)	249/1347 (18.5)	855/6743 (12.7)
16–59	120/2984 (4.0)	104/2360 (4.4)	108/2040 (5.3)	87/2474 (3.5)	147/2830 (5.2)	153/2682 (5.7)	719/15,370 (4.7)
60<	71/3482 (2.0)	54/3888 (1.4)	52/3714 (1.4)	32/4535 (0.7)	113/6025 (1.9)	121/5111 (2.4)	443/26,755 (1.7)
Total	819/10,215 (8.0)	556/9380 (5.9)	966/10,106 (9.6)	1038/11,555 (9.0)	1130/13,886 (8.1)	1143/12,017 (9.5)	5652/67,159 (8.4)

Analysis of norovirus detection rates by year revealed some fluctuations over the study period. In 2019, the detection rate was 8.0% (819/10,215), which decreased significantly to 5.9% (556/9380) in 2020, coinciding with the onset of the COVID-19 pandemic ($p < 0.001$). The detection rate peaked at 9.6% in 2021 and subsequently remained at 9.0% in 2022, 8.1% in 2023, and 9.5% in 2024, showing a trend toward recovery to the pre-pandemic level observed in 2019. Monthly detection patterns are shown in Figure 1. The highest monthly detection rate was observed in January 2024 (25.8%), whereas the lowest was in September 2023 (0.5%). Detection rates exceeding 20% were predominantly observed in January–February, while lower rates (~5%) were noted during the summer and fall months (June–October). Notably, in 2022, detection rates began to rise sharply from May, reaching 21.5% in June. The Cochran–Armitage test confirmed a statistically significant upward trend in detection rates from 2020–2024 ($p < 0.01$), supporting the observation of a post-pandemic resurgence of norovirus.

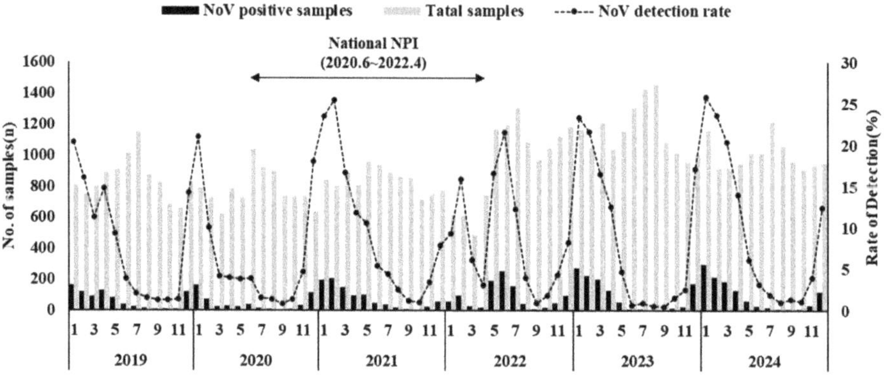

Figure 1. Temporal trends in norovirus detection rates in South Korea during 2019–2024. Monthly detection rates are shown for acute gastroenteritis surveillance. Non-pharmaceutical COVID-19 interventions (social distancing, mask wearing, and school closures) were implemented from June 2020 to April 2022 and are indicated on the timeline.

3.2. Norovirus Genotyping (G and P Type)

Genotype analysis was performed on norovirus-positive samples from children aged ≤5 years. Among these samples, 72.4% (2633/3635) were successfully amplified by RT-PCR and sequenced. When analyzed by year, sequencing success rates for retrospectively analyzed samples from 2019, 2020, and 2021 were 66.6% (353/530), 55.6% (180/324), and 55.4% (353/637), respectively. In contrast, samples subjected to dual typing immediately after norovirus detection in 2022, 2023, and 2024 showed relatively higher sequencing success rates of 83.2% (668/803), 81.7% (589/721), and 79.0% (490/620), respectively. Among all successfully sequenced samples (n = 2633), a total of 31 genotypes were identified, including 9 GI and 22 GII genotypes. The distribution of the seven most frequent genotypes is shown in Figure 2A. Across both GI and GII genogroups, the most frequently detected genotype was GII.4[P31], accounting for 37.1% (977/2633) of sequences, followed by GII.4[P16] (26.4%, n = 695), GII.2[P16] (10.2%, n = 268), GII.3[P12] (7.9%, n = 208), and GII.6[P7] (5.6%, n = 148).

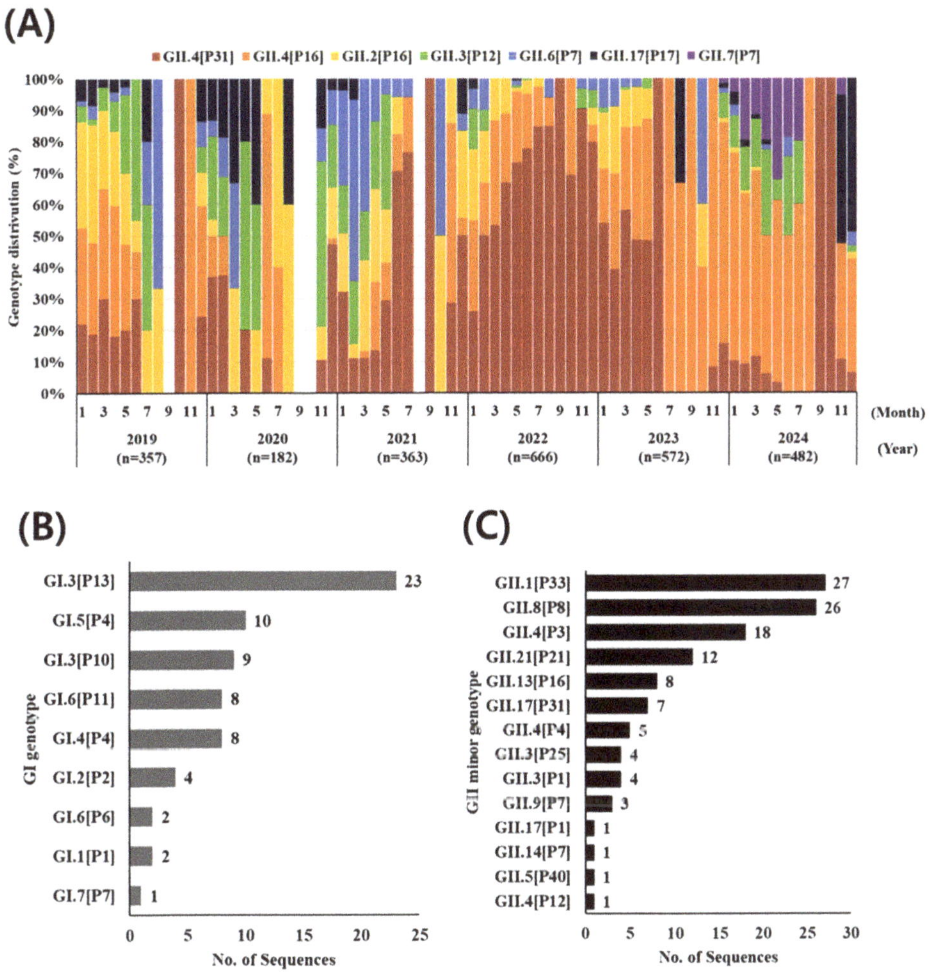

Figure 2. Distribution of norovirus genotypes in South Korea during 2019–2024. (**A**) Annual distribution of major genotypes (2019–2021 analyzed retrospectively). (**B**) Distribution of GI genotypes detected. (**C**) Minor GII genotypes detected at ≤2% frequency. Genotyping was based on dual analysis of the RdRp–VP1 junction.

During 2019–2021, multiple genotypes were detected at relatively comparable frequencies of approximately 20%. In 2019, GII.4[P16] (29.5%), GII.2[P16] (23.2%), and GII.4[P31] (20.1%) together accounted for more than 70% of all cases. In 2020, the predominant genotype was GII.4[P31] (27.8%), followed by GII.3[P12] (21.7%), indicating a shift from the previous year. In 2021, GII.4[P31] remained predominant (23.2%), but GII.6[P7] (20.4%) emerged as the second most frequent genotype. However, in 2022, GII.4[P31] overwhelmingly dominated the entire year, accounting for 72.9% of all detections, followed by GII.4[P16] (16.2%), whereas other genotypes that had been more common in previous years, such as GII.3[P12], GII.6[P7], and GII.17[P17] declined substantially. In 2023, GII.4[P31] continued to predominate during the first half of the year but was superseded by GII.4[P16] in the second half. This predominance of GII.4[P16] persisted into the first half of 2024, during which GII.3[P12] also re-emerged. In the latter half of 2024, a notable increase in GII.7[P7], which had not been observed in previous years, was detected ($n = 59$). Subsequently, from November 2024 onward, GII.17[P17] markedly increased and became the predominant genotype. This sharp increase illustrates a clear genotype replacement event, in which GII.17[P17] rapidly displaced GII.4-associated strains within a single winter season.

A total of 67 samples from the GI group were successfully genotyped during the study period (Figure 2B). The most frequently detected genotype was GI.3[P13] ($n = 23$), with an annual average of six cases (range: 1–8), peaking at eight cases in 2021. The second most common genotype was GI.5[P4] ($n = 10$), seven cases of which were concentrated in 2021. GI.3[P10] ($n = 9$) was also identified, with most detections ($n = 8$) occurring in 2023, suggesting that this genotype exhibited a temporally restricted outbreak pattern. Additional GI genotypes, along with relatively rare GII genotypes ($\leq$2% of total detections), are presented in Figure 2C. Although detected at low overall frequencies, these minor genotypes were temporally clustered, indicating that they may represent localized outbreaks or introductions from external sources. Their sporadic appearance underscores the need for sensitive surveillance capable of capturing low-level but epidemiologically relevant events.

4. Discussion

Norovirus is one of the most important viral agents causing acute gastroenteritis (AGE) worldwide. In Korea, surveillance of five major viral pathogens (norovirus, group A rotavirus, enteric adenovirus, astrovirus, and sapovirus) has consistently demonstrated the highest detection rates for norovirus [24]. In the present study, we analyzed nationwide data over a six-year period, including the COVID-19 pandemic, to investigate the epidemiological trends and genotype distribution of noroviruses, and further characterized the circulating strains using G–P dual typing. In the present study, the average detection rate of norovirus among children aged $\leq$ 5 years was 19.9% (range: 14.3–23.2%) during 2019–2024, which was slightly higher than the previously reported average detection rate of 15.2% (range: 11.8–18.9%) during 2013–2019 [25]. When considering all age groups, the detection rate in 2020 decreased significantly compared with 2019, coinciding with the onset of the COVID-19 pandemic in Korea (February 2020) and the implementation of strict social distancing and public health measures in April of the same year. Previous studies have also reported that the COVID-19 pandemic influenced the transmission of noroviruses [21,26–29]. With the introduction of NPIs, including social distancing, mask wearing, and the closure of schools and childcare facilities, the seasonal epidemic pattern of norovirus was altered, and a temporary sharp decline in detection rates was observed [7,19].

From 2021 onward, the detection rate gradually increased, returning to levels comparable to those observed in 2019. Notably, during the summer of 2022, the detection rate rose to substantially higher levels than the seasonal average, coinciding with the relaxation of social distancing stipulations and other public health measures as Korea entered the post-pandemic phase. This finding is consistent with those of previous reports describing atypical timing and scale of norovirus resurgences in several regions following the easing of public health restrictions [7,19,20]. Although a direct causal relationship between norovirus detection rates and COVID-19 cannot be established, our findings—together with those of earlier studies—suggest that stringent NPIs implemented during the early phase of the pandemic likely contributed to the suppression of norovirus and other water- and foodborne viral epidemics in Korea. Norovirus undergoes continuous genotype replacement, which is one of the major challenges for vaccine development. To date, no licensed vaccine is available, and questions remain regarding the duration of immunity and the extent of cross-protection among different genotypes [1,30]. The identification of predominant strains such as GII.4[P31], GII.4[P16], and the emerging GII.17[P17] provides critical evidence for prioritizing candidate antigens for vaccine development and assessing the breadth of cross-protective immunity in future vaccine trials. In this study, we performed genotyping analysis of positive samples obtained from children aged ≤5 years. This age group had the highest proportion of norovirus-positive cases, ensuring both representativeness of the dataset and practicality in terms of analytical efficiency and resource allocation. Sequencing success was lower in 2019–2021 due to retrospective typing from archived material (likely RNA degradation), whereas immediate dual typing since 2022 improved success. Although incomplete sequencing may introduce minor bias, the genotyped subset mirrored the temporal distribution of all positives, making substantial distortion of predominant genotype rankings unlikely.

According to our findings, the predominant genotypes detected in Korea were GII.4[P31] and GII.4[P16], which is consistent with globally reported circulating strains [1,7,20]. For example, in Shanghai, China, GII.4 Sydney[P31] and GII.3[P12] were the major genotypes detected between 2018 and 2021, with evidence of genotype replacement occurring over time [20]. In Brazil, multiple genotypes were detected even during the COVID-19 pandemic, and a re-emergence of GII.4 variants was reported in the post-pandemic period [7]. According to data analyzed from NoroSurv, the prevalence of the GII.17 genotype, which had previously been uncommon, increased in 2025 following the end of the COVID-19 pandemic [31]. Similarly, in Korea, we observed a marked increase in the detection of GII.17[P17] during the winter of late 2024. This replacement event highlights the dynamic nature of norovirus evolution and suggests that novel genotypes may rapidly establish dominance under favorable epidemiological conditions, underscoring the necessity of continuous real-time monitoring.

These findings highlight the importance of cross-country comparisons and long-term genomic surveillance for monitoring shifts in predominant genotypes [2,7,32]. In addition, although some genotypes showed low overall detection rates across the study period, they were concentrated in specific years, suggesting the possibility of transient or localized outbreaks. Given that several of these minor genotypes have been reported in neighboring countries during similar timeframes, their detection in Korea may also reflect cross-border transmissions, further emphasizing the importance of global data sharing. Therefore, continuous monitoring of circulation patterns is necessary, even for genotypes with low detection frequencies.

Despite these important findings, this study has several limitations that should be acknowledged. First, genotype analysis was restricted to samples from children aged ≤5 years, which may not fully represent genotype circulation across the entire population. Second, our sequencing strategy targeted only the RdRp–VP1 junction, which provides robust dual typing and enables detection of recombinant events but does not offer sufficient resolution for variant-level designation. As variant-defining substitutions in GII.4 lineages are distributed across the VP1, particularly within the P2 subdomain, full-length VP1 or whole-genome sequencing would be required to confidently distinguish Sydney_2012 and emerging descendant variants. To avoid over-interpretation, genotypes were therefore reported at the G-P typing level (e.g., GII.4[P31], GII.4[P16]), and Sydney_2012-like clustering was noted only where extended VP1 information was available. Future sequencing efforts incorporating full-length VP1 or whole genomes would allow a more detailed characterization of recombination dynamics and variant evolution. Additionally, the consistently higher detection rates in certain provinces, such as Gwangju, compared with persistently low rates in regions such as Chungbuk and Jeju, suggest geographic heterogeneity in transmission dynamics. These differences may reflect variations in population density, healthcare-seeking behavior, or environmental factors, and warrant further investigation. Because our data comes from a sentinel network with region-specific participation, differences in hospital mix and patient age structure may influence specimen volumes and positivity. Therefore, regional detection rates reported here should be interpreted with caution and may not directly mirror true community incidence.

Future studies should expand surveillance to include broader age groups and apply whole-genome sequencing to obtain a more comprehensive understanding of norovirus genetic diversity. In addition, strengthening data sharing through international surveillance platforms such as NoroSurv will be crucial for integrating national findings with global trends. Linking molecular epidemiology with clinical and immunological data will further contribute to vaccine development and public health preparedness. Strengthening national surveillance capacity, including facilitating timely data sharing with international platforms, will be critical for early warning of emerging variants and for guiding evidence-based public health interventions in Korea.

5. Conclusions

This study analyzed the genotype distribution and detection trends of noroviruses in Korea over the past six years, encompassing both the pre- and post-COVID-19 pandemic periods, using nationwide surveillance data and a dual typing approach. By integrating dual genotyping with long-term nationwide data, this study provides one of the most comprehensive molecular epidemiological datasets on noroviruses in Korea to date. The emergence of novel genotypes such as GII.17[P17] underscores the need to reconsider vaccine targets and highlights the importance of variant monitoring systems. These insights will be instrumental for informing vaccine candidate selection and evaluating the extent of cross-protective immunity across genotypes. Our findings contribute to integrating national epidemiological data into global surveillance trends and serve as valuable evidence for the development of future public health policies. Ongoing genomic monitoring, coupled with timely international data sharing, will be critical for early warning of emerging variants and for aligning Korea's surveillance capacity with global networks. Future research should incorporate whole-genome sequencing, antigenic characterization, and integration with clinical severity data to better understand viral evolution and host–virus interactions, thereby supporting more effective vaccine development and preparedness strategies.

Supplementary Materials: The following supporting information can be downloaded at: https://www.mdpi.com/article/10.3390/v17121572/s1, Table S1: Regional distribution of norovirus-positive samples and detection rates among acute gastroenteritis cases, South Ko-rea during 2019–2024.

Author Contributions: Conceptualization, D.-Y.L.; Methodology, Y.J.; Validation, M.L.; Formal analysis, S.-R.C.; Resources, S.-R.C., Y.J. and D.-Y.L.; Data curation, M.L., S.-R.C., Y.J. and D.-Y.L.; Writing—original draft, M.L.; Writing—review & editing, S.-W.P.; Visualization, M.L.; Supervision, M.-G.H. and S.-W.P.; Project administration, M.-G.H. and S.-W.P.; Funding acquisition, M.-G.H. and S.-W.P. All authors have read and agreed to the published version of the manuscript.

Funding: This study was supported by intramural funds (Grant No. 6332-304) from the Korea Disease Control and Prevention Agency (KDCA).

Institutional Review Board Statement: In accordance with institutional policy, analyses conducted for routine national public health surveillance are not considered human-subjects research. Therefore, institutional review board approval was not required for this study.

Informed Consent Statement: Patient consent was waived because anonymized stool specimens collected for routine national public health surveillance were used. No patient-identifiable information was included, and informed consent was not required.

Data Availability Statement: The original contributions presented in this study are included in the article and its Supplementary Material. In addition, a non-redundant, genotype-representative subset of the nucleotide sequence data generated in this study has been deposited in GenBank under accession numbers [PX598973-PX598992, PX599239-PX599306, PX599383-PX599529, PX599585-PX599634, PX599732-PX599767, PX599773-PX599997]. Further inquiries, including access to additional sequence data, can be directed to the corresponding author.

Acknowledgments: We thank the staff of the EnterNet-Korea sentinel hospitals and laboratories for their efforts in sample collection and diagnostics.

Conflicts of Interest: The authors declare no conflicts of interest.

References

1. Carlson, K.B.; Dilley, A.; O'Grady, T.; Johnson, J.A.; Lopman, B.; Viscidi, E. A narrative review of norovirus epidemiology, biology, and challenges to vaccine development. *npj Vaccines* **2016**, *7*, 870. [CrossRef] [PubMed]
2. Farahmand, M.; Moghoofei, M.; Dorost, A.; Shoja, Z.; Ghorbani, S.; Kiani, S.J.; Khales, P.; Esteghamati, A.; Sayyahfar, S.; Jafarzadeh, M.; et al. Global prevalence and genotype distribution of norovirus infection in children with gastroenteritis: A meta-analysis on 6 years of research from 2015 to 2020. *Rev. Med Virol.* **2022**, 3, e94–e104. [CrossRef] [PubMed]
3. Patel, M.M.; Hall, A.J.; Vinjé, J.; Parashar, U.D. Noroviruses: A comprehensive review. *J. Clin. Virol.* **2009**, *44*, 1–8. [CrossRef] [PubMed]
4. Lopman, B.A.; Steele, D.; Kirkwood, C.D.; Parashar, U.D. The vast and varied global burden of norovirus: Prospects for prevention and control. *PLoS Med.* **2016**, *13*, e1001999. [CrossRef]
5. Hall, A.J.; Lopman, B.A.; Payne, D.C.; Patel, M.M.; Gastanaduy, P.A.; Vinjé, J.; Parashar, U.D. Norovirus disease in the United States. *Emerg. Infect. Dis.* **2013**, *19*, 1198–1205. [CrossRef]
6. de Graaf, M.; van Beek, J.; Koopmans, M. Human norovirus transmission and evolution in a changing world. *Nat. Rev. Microbiol.* **2016**, *14*, 421–433. [CrossRef]
7. Sarmento, S.K.; de Andrade, J.D.S.R.; Malta, F.C.; Fialho, A.M.; Mello, M.D.S.; Burlandy, F.M.; Fumian, T.M. Norovirus Epidemiology and Genotype Circulation during the COVID-19 Pandemic in Brazil, 2019–2022. *Pathogens* **2024**, *13*, 3. [CrossRef]
8. Green, K. Caliciviridae: The Noroviruses. In *Fields Virology*, 6th ed.; Knipe, D.M., Howley, P.M., Eds.; Lippincott Williams & Wilkins: Philadelphia, PA, USA, 2013; pp. 582–608.
9. Cannon, J.L.; Bonifacio, J.; Bucardo, F.; Buesa, J.; Bruggink, L.; Chan, M.C.W.; Fumian, T.M.; Giri, S.; Gonzalez, M.D.; Hewitt, J.; et al. Global Trends in Norovirus Genotype Distribution among Children with Acute Gastroenteritis. *Emerg. Infect. Dis.* **2021**, *27*, 1438–1445. [CrossRef]
10. Chhabra, P.; de Graaf, M.; Parra, G.I.; Chan, M.C.; Green, K.; Martella, V.; Wang, Q.; White, P.A.; Katayama, K.; Vennema, H.; et al. Updated classification of norovirus genogroups and genotypes. *J. Gen. Virol.* **2019**, *100*, 1393–1406. [CrossRef]
11. Siebenga, J.J.; Vennema, H.; Zheng, D.P.; Vinjé, J.; Lee, B.E.; Pang, X.L.; Ho, E.C.; Lim, W.; Choudekar, A.; Broor, S.; et al. Norovirus illness is a global problem: Emergence and spread of norovirus GII.4 variants, 2001–2007. *J. Infect. Dis.* **2009**, *200*, 802–812. [CrossRef]
12. Hernandez, J.M.; Silva, L.D.; Sousa Junior, E.C.; Cardoso, J.F.; Reymão, T.K.A.; Portela, A.C.R.; de Lima, C.P.S.; Teixeira, D.M.; Lucena, M.S.S.; Nunes, M.R.T.; et al. Evolutionary and Molecular Analysis of Complete Genome Sequences of Norovirus from Brazil: Emerging Recombinant Strain GII.P16/GII.4. *Front. Microbiol.* **2020**, *11*, 1870. [CrossRef] [PubMed]
13. Kroneman, A.; Vega, E.; Vennema, H.; Vinjé, J.; White, P.A.; Hansman, G.; Green, K.; Martella, V.; Katayama, K.; Koopmans, M. Proposal for a unified norovirus nomenclature and genotyping. *Arch. Virol.* **2013**, *158*, 2059–2068. [CrossRef]
14. CDC. CaliciNet Surveillance Network. CDC Norovirus (Reporting & Surveillance). 2024. Available online: https://www.cdc.gov/norovirus/php/reporting/calicinet.html (accessed on 22 August 2025).
15. Vega, E.; Barclay, L.; Gregoricus, N.; Williams, K.; Lee, D.; Vinjé, J. Novel surveillance network for norovirus gastroenteritis outbreaks, United States. *Emerg. Infect. Dis.* **2011**, *17*, 1389–1395. [CrossRef] [PubMed]

16. Kroneman, A.; Vennema, H.; Deforche, K.; v d Avoort, H.; Penaranda, S.; Oberste, M.S.; Vinjé, J.; Koopmans, M. An automated genotyping tool for enteroviruses and noroviruses. *J. Clin. Virol.* **2011**, *51*, 121–125. [CrossRef] [PubMed]
17. Eden, J.S.; Tanaka, M.M.; Boni, M.F.; Rawlinson, W.D.; White, P.A. Recombination within the pandemic norovirus GII.4 lineage. *J. Virol.* **2013**, *87*, 6270–6282. [CrossRef]
18. Mans, J.; Armah, G.E.; Steele, A.D.; Taylor, M.B. Norovirus epidemiology in Africa: A review. *PLoS ONE* **2016**, *11*, e0146280. [CrossRef]
19. Li, J.; Wang, B.; He, X.; Li, Z.; Sun, L.; Li, W.; Bai, G. Epidemiological characteristics of norovirus infection in pediatric patients during the COVID-19 pandemic. *J. Med. Virol.* **2023**, *95*, e28874. [CrossRef]
20. Lu, L.; Ao, Y.; Jia, R.; Zhong, H.; Liu, P.; Xu, M.; Su, L.; Cao, L.; Xu, J. Changing predominance of norovirus strains in children with acute gastroenteritis in Shanghai, 2018–2021. *Virol. Sin.* **2023**, *38*, 671–679. [CrossRef]
21. Liu, P.; Xu, M.; Lu, L.; Ma, A.; Cao, L.; Su, L.; Dong, N.; Jia, R.; Zhu, X.; Xu, J. The Changing Pattern of Common Respiratory and Enteric Viruses among Outpatient Children in Shanghai, China: Two Years of the COVID-19 Pandemic. *J. Med. Virol.* **2022**, *94*, 4696–4703. [CrossRef]
22. Kraay, A.N.M.; Han, P.; Kambhampati, A.; Wikswo, M.E.; Mirza, S.A.; Lopman, B.A. Impact of Nonpharmaceutical Interventions for Severe Acute Respiratory Syndrome Coronavirus 2 on Norovirus Outbreaks: An Analysis of Outbreaks Reported By 9 US States. *J. Infect. Dis.* **2021**, *224*, 9–13. [CrossRef]
23. Kojima, S.; Kageyama, T.; Fukushi, S.; Hoshino, F.B.; Shinohara, M.; Uchida, K.; Natori, K.; Takeda, N.; Katayama, K. Genogroup-specific PCR primers for detection of Norwalk-like viruses. *J. Virol. Methods* **2002**, *100*, 107–114. [CrossRef] [PubMed]
24. Lee, M.; Jo, Y.; Park, S.-W.; Han, M.-G. Recent Trends in the Circulation of Viruses Causing Acute Gastroenteritis in the Republic of Korea, 2019–2023. *Public Health Wkly. Rep.* **2024**, *17*, 1786–1801. [CrossRef]
25. Cho, S.-R.; Chae, S.-J.; Jung, S.; Choi, W.; Han, M.-G.; Yoo, C.-K.; Lee, D.-Y. Trends in acute viral gastroenteritis among children aged ≤5 years through the national surveillance system in South Korea, 2013–2019. *J. Med. Virol.* **2021**, *93*, 4875–4882. [CrossRef] [PubMed]
26. Nachamkin, I.; Richard-Greenblatt, M.; Yu, M.; Bui, H. Reduction in Sporadic Norovirus Infections Following the Start of the COVID-19 Pandemic, 2019–2020, Philadelphia. *Infect. Dis. Ther.* **2021**, *10*, 1793–1798. [CrossRef]
27. Lennon, R.P.; Griffin, C.; Miller, E.L.; Dong, H.; Rabago, D.; Zgierska, A.E. Norovirus Infections Drop 49% in the United States with Strict COVID-19 Public Health Interventions. *Acta Med. Acad.* **2020**, *49*, 278–280. [CrossRef]
28. Chan, M.C. Return of Norovirus and Rotavirus Activity in Winter 2020–21 in City with Strict COVID-19 Control Strategy, China. *Emerg. Infect. Dis.* **2022**, *28*, 713–716. [CrossRef]
29. Jacobsen, S.; Faber, M.; Altmann, B.; Mas Marques, A.; Bock, C.T.; Niendorf, S. Impact of the COVID-19 pandemic on norovirus circulation in Germany. *Int. J. Med. Microbiol.* **2024**, *314*, 151600. [CrossRef]
30. Atmar, R.L.; Bernstein, D.I.; Lyon, G.M.; Treanor, J.J.; Al-Ibrahim, M.S.; Graham, D.Y.; Vinjé, J.; Jiang, X.; Gregoricus, N.; Frenck, R.W.; et al. Serological correlates of protection against a GII.4 norovirus. *Clin. Vaccine Immunol.* **2015**, *22*, 923–929. [CrossRef]
31. Vinjé, J. Advances in laboratory methods for detection and typing of norovirus. *J. Clin. Microbiol.* **2015**, *53*, 373–381. [CrossRef]
32. Kendra, J.A.; Tohma, K.; Parra, G.I. Global and regional circulation trends of norovirus genotypes and recombinants, 1995–2019: A comprehensive review of sequences from public databases. *Rev. Med. Virol.* **2022**, *32*, e2354. [CrossRef]

viruses

MDPI

Brief Report

Delayed Emergence of Norovirus GII.17 in Finland: Foodborne Outbreaks Reported During the 2024/25 Season

Haider Al-Hello [1,2,*], Ruska Rimhanen-Finne [1] and Carita Savolainen-Kopra [1]

[1] Department of Public Health, National Institute for Health and Welfare, 00300 Helsinki, Finland; ruska.rimhanen-finne@thl.fi (R.R.-F.); carita.savolainen-kopra@thl.fi (C.S.-K.)
[2] Faculty of Dentistry, University of Cordoba, Najaf 54001, Iraq
* Correspondence: haider.al-hello@thl.fi

Abstract

During the 2024/25 season, Finland experienced a delayed emergence of norovirus genotype GII.17, which had already become prevalent in several European countries and the United States during the previous season, 2023/24. In Finland, GII.17 was confirmed in three foodborne outbreaks and five sporadic cases, marking the highest number of detections to date. These cases were geographically distributed across southern, western, and northern Finland, indicating widespread circulation. Retrospective analysis of national surveillance data from 2014 to 2025 revealed that GII.17 had been detected sporadically in earlier years but never at this scale. The emergence of GII.17 coincided with a continued presence of GII.4 [P16], the previously dominant genotype. Phylogenetic analysis showed that Finnish GII.17 strains clustered with recent international strains, suggesting introduction from abroad. The findings highlight the importance of sustained genotyping and international surveillance to detect emerging norovirus variants and inform public health preparedness in Finland.

Keywords: norovirus; GII.17; retrospective analysis; phylogenetic analysis

1. Introduction

Human norovirus is the leading cause of acute gastroenteritis worldwide, responsible for an estimated 685 million cases annually, including 200 million among children under five [1]. The virus contributes to approximately 200,000 deaths each year, with the highest burden in low-income countries [1]. Beyond its health impact, norovirus imposes a significant economic burden, estimated at USD 60 billion globally due to healthcare costs and productivity losses [1]. In Finland, norovirus is a major cause of gastroenteritis outbreaks, particularly in institutional settings such as long-term care facilities and schools. Norovirus genotyping is conducted as a statutory part of food- and waterborne outbreak investigations [2]. Viruses in person-to-person transmissions are not routinely genotyped; instead, they are typically included in collaborative research studies. Norovirus genotyping is based on sequencing specific regions of the viral genome, particularly the capsid gene (VP1) and the RNA-dependent RNA polymerase (RdRp) gene [3]. These sequences are then compared to the typing tools implemented by the NoroNet to determine the genotype [4].

Norovirus genotype GII.17 has recently gained attention due to its rapid emergence and spread in several regions, occasionally surpassing the historically dominant GII.4 strains. Unlike earlier genotypes, GII.17 exhibits distinct amino acid substitutions in the capsid protein, particularly in the P2 subdomain, which influence its antigenic properties and receptor binding affinity. These changes may enhance immune evasion and broaden host susceptibility [5,6].

In Finland, laboratory-confirmed norovirus infections are mandatorily reported to the Finnish Infectious Diseases Register (FIDR) as part of a surveillance system coordinated by the Finnish Institute for Health and Welfare (THL). The reporting is based on nucleic acid detection methods, primarily RT-PCR, which identify human norovirus genogroups GI and GII from stool specimens. The analysis of national norovirus surveillance data from the Finnish Infectious Disease Registry (FIDR) between 2014 and 2025 reveals a biennial norovirus notification pattern with higher case numbers observed every other year (Figure 1). In the three seasons during and following the COVID-19 pandemic (2021/22, 2022/23 and 2023/24), the number of norovirus notifications resembled the levels typically seen during pre-pandemic norovirus epidemic years (2016/17 and 2018/19).

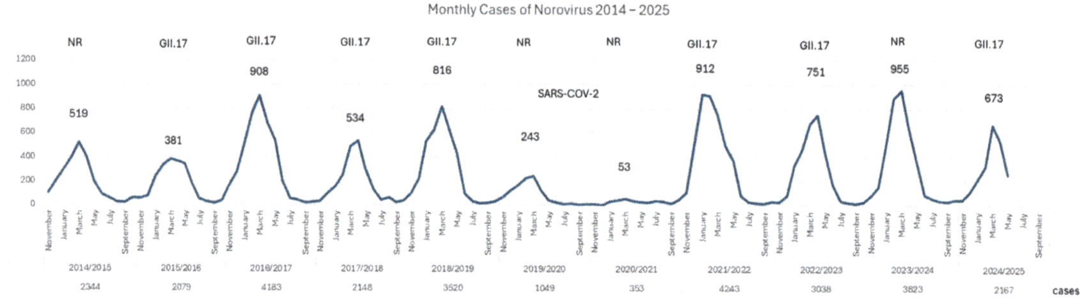

Figure 1. Monthly reported norovirus cases in Finland from the 2015/16 to 2024/25 seasons. This figure illustrates a biennial pattern of norovirus epidemics in Finland, with notable peaks in the 2016/17, 2018/19, 2021/22, and 2023/24 seasons. The numbers on the peaks indicate the total number of cases at each peak. The total number of cases for the entire season is mentioned below. GII.17 refers to the years in which this genotype was detected. A significant decline in cases is observed during the COVID-19 pandemic years (2019/20 and 2020/21); three years after the pandemic, norovirus case numbers were like those seen in norovirus epidemic years before the pandemic began. Notably, GII.17 norovirus has been detected in both high-incidence and low-incidence seasons, indicating its persistent circulation regardless of overall epidemic intensity. The 2024/25 season marks the highest number of GII.17 detections to date, in both outbreaks and sporadic cases. NR = no record.

During the 2023/24 season, Finland participated in enhanced norovirus surveillance alongside other European countries and the USA [7]. A notable increase in GII.17 norovirus outbreaks and sporadic cases occurred in Austria, Germany, France, Ireland, the Netherlands, England, and the United States. This rise in GII.17 prevalence coincided with a decline in the previously dominant GII.4 genotype, with GII.17 accounting for 17% to 64% of all GII detections in the affected countries. In Finland, however, no GII.17 noroviruses were detected.

2. Materials and Methods

2.1. Surveillance and Case Reporting

Norovirus infections in Finland are mandatorily reported to the National Infectious Diseases Register (NIDR), coordinated by the Finnish Institute for Health and Welfare (THL). Reporting is based on nucleic acid detection methods, primarily reverse-transcription polymerase chain reaction (RT-PCR), which identify norovirus genogroups GI and GII from stool specimens.

2.2. Outbreak Surveillance

In Finland, the municipal food- and waterborne outbreak investigation groups notify suspected norovirus outbreaks to the Finnish Food and Waterborne Outbreak Registry (FWOR) [2]. We reviewed the FWOR notifications from the 2014/15 to 2024/25 seasons, in order to better understand the emergence of GII.17 in Finland.

2.3. Sample Selection and Genotyping

Stool specimens from outbreak-related and sporadic cases were collected and submitted for genotyping. Sporadic cases were selected from diagnostic laboratories across Finland to monitor the prevalence of noroviruses including GII.17 outside of FWOs. NoV RNA was extracted using the QIAamp Viral RNA Mini QIAcube Kit (Qiagen, Hilden, Germany) or Chemagic Viral DNA/RNA 300 Kit H96 (PerkinElmer, Inc., Waltham, MA, USA). Norovirus genotyping was conducted by sequencing regions of the viral genome from the capsid gene (VP1) and the RNA-dependent RNA polymerase (RdRp) gene using a one-step RT-PCR kit (Qiagen) according to Vinjé et al. (2004) [3]. Sequences were analyzed using Geneious 6.0.5 software [8] and Sequencher version 5.4.6 DNA sequence analysis software (Gene Codes Corporation, Ann Arbor, MI, USA). The sequences were then compared with other isolates using the NoroNet typing tool (accessed on 18 November 2025 https://mpf.rivm.nl/mpf/norovirus/typingtool/) to determine the genotype.

2.4. Phylogenetic Analysis

Phylogenetic trees were constructed using MEGA 12 software [9], applying the Tamura–Nei model [10] with 1000 bootstrap replications. Separate trees were generated for the capsid (VP1) and polymerase (RdRp) regions to assess genetic relationships between Finnish GII.17 strains and global reference sequences. The analysis included sequences from outbreaks and sporadic cases detected during the 2024/25 season. Finnish sequences from the preceding season were also included. All sequences have been uploaded to GenBank under accession numbers PV973171–PV973223.

2.5. Ethical Considerations

All data used in this study were collected as part of statutory public health surveillance and outbreak investigations. No personal identifiers were included, and ethical approval was not required for this analysis.

3. Results

While GII.17 was first detected in Finland in the 2015/16 season (Table 1), it remained rare and sporadic in subsequent years, with isolated detections in both outbreak-related and sporadic cases. The sporadic cases were selected to monitor the prevalence of the GII.17 strain in non-FWOs and requested from diagnostic laboratories across Finland.

During the 2024/25 season, FWOR contained 98 outbreak notifications, of which 41 (42%) were suspected to be caused by norovirus (Table 1). Noroviruses from four outbreaks were genotyped, and GII.17 was confirmed in three of them, with an estimated 164 cases. The suspected sources were dining outside the home and person-to-person transmission. Of the twelve sporadic cases, five were genotyped as GII.17. The outbreaks occurred in southern, western, and northern Finland, while the sporadic cases were reported in the south and west. This suggests that GII.17 is circulating across the entire country.

Table 1. Number of food- and waterborne outbreak notifications and norovirus findings in Finland during norovirus seasons, 2014–2025.

Season	Number of Notified Outbreaks	Number of Outbreaks in Which Norovirus Is the Suspected Cause	Number of Outbreaks/ Sporadic Cases with Genotyped Noroviruses	Number of Outbreaks/Sporadic Cases with Confirmed GII.17 Finding
2014/15	67	20	10 + 48 *	NR
2015/16	80	34	24 + 20 *	2
2016/17	63	22	7 + 40 *	1 + 1 *
2017/18	80	30	21 + 37 *	4
2018/19	93	35	12 + 66 *	4 + 5 *
2019/20	72	20	4 + 27 *	NR
2020/21	58	4	1	NR
2021/22	89	26	12	1
2022/23	89	26	11 + 34 *	1 + 2 *
2023/24	108	33	9 + 23 *	NR
2024/25	98	41	4 + 12 *	3 + 5 *

Season starts in July and ends in June the subsequent year. NR stands for no record. * Sporadic case.

In Finland, GII.17 norovirus has been detected in both high-incidence and low-incidence years, indicating that its circulation is not strictly dependent on overall epidemic intensity. Despite the sharp decline in total human norovirus cases during the pandemic years (2019/20 and 2020/21), GII.17 re-emerged post-pandemic and was most frequently detected in the 2024/25 season, in both outbreaks and sporadic cases.

Finnish isolates from the 2024/25 season are highlighted in red, while other Finnish isolates are shown in blue. Maximum-likelihood phylogenetic trees were computed within MEGA 12 [9] using Tamura–Nei [10] with 1000 bootstrap replications. The Finnish sequence accession numbers are as follows: PV973171–PV973223; more details are provided in Supplementary Table S1.

The phylogenetic tree in Figure 2A based on the capsid gene (VP1) of GII.17 norovirus strains illustrates the genetic relationships between Finnish GII.17 sequences and global reference strains (Figure 2A). Sequences from Finland, including those recently found, cluster closely with strains from recent years (2023–2025), suggesting that the currently circulating GII.17 strains in Finland are part of the globally emerging lineage that has evolved from earlier variants first detected around 2015 and 2017.

The phylogenetic tree of the polymerase region (GII.P17) is like the VP1 phylogenetic tree; Finnish sequences from 2025 also cluster with recent international strains, indicating co-evolution of the polymerase and capsid regions. The presence of closely related sequences in both trees supports the conclusion that the current GII.17 viruses circulating in Finland are genetically like those causing outbreaks in other parts of the world.

(**A**)

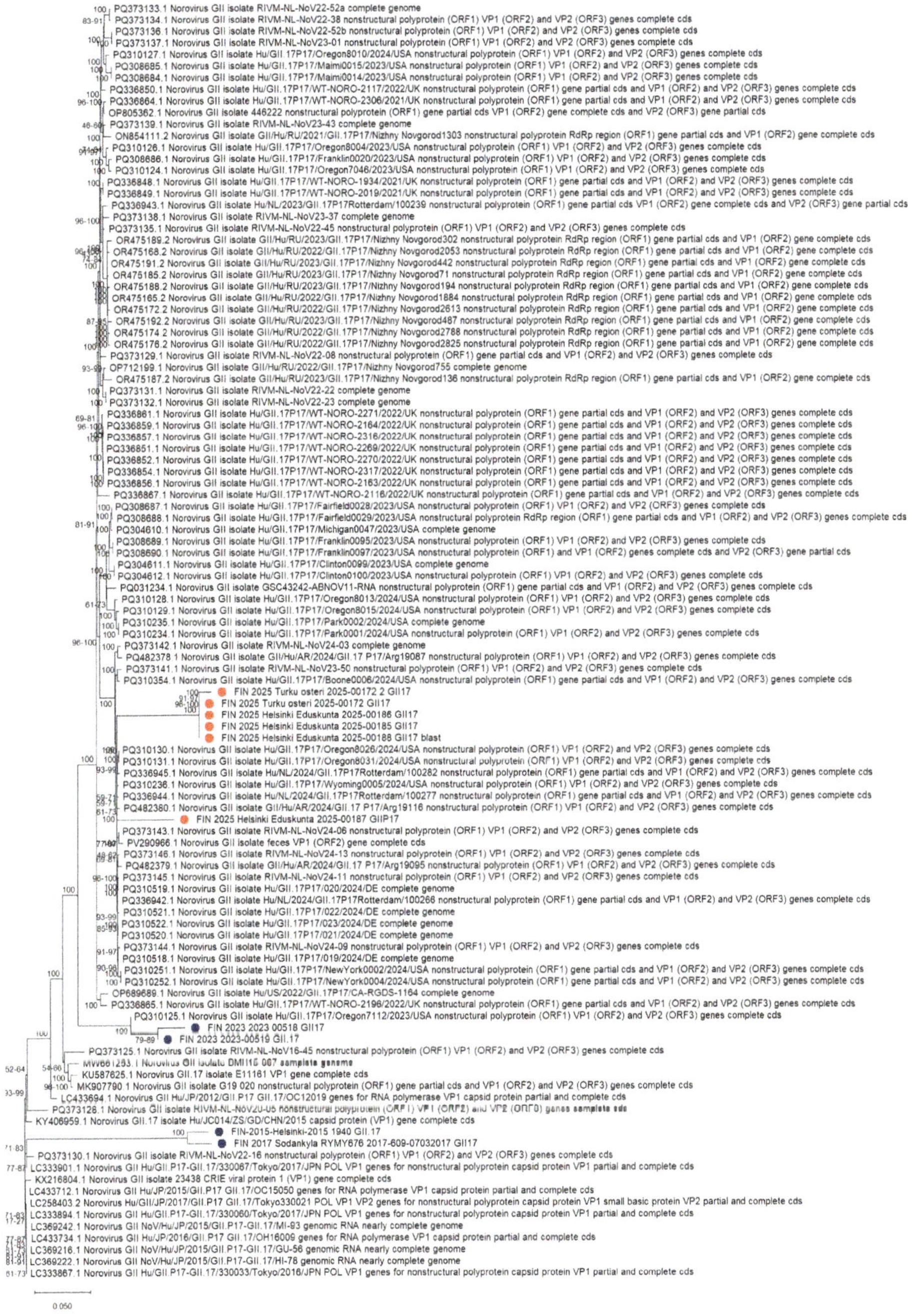

Figure 2. *Cont.*

(**B**)

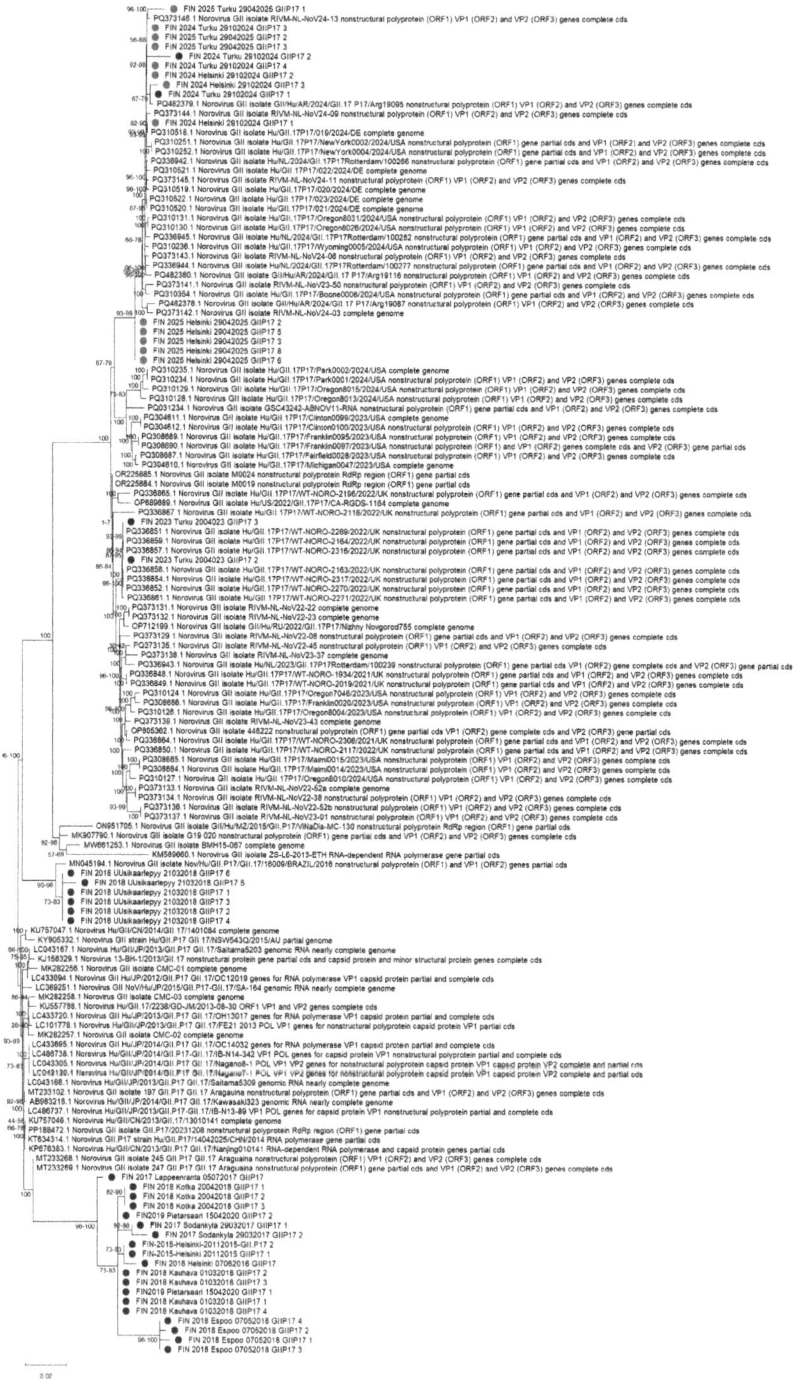

Figure 2. (**A**) Phylogenetic analysis of ten Finnish GII.17 VP1 sequences (200–290 bp) and 77 corresponding global sequences. (**B**) Phylogenetic analysis of 42 Finnish GII.P17 polymerase sequences (170–260 bp) and 100 corresponding global sequences.

4. Discussion

Norovirus GII.17 emerged later in Finland than in Central Europe and Russia, where the virus had already caused widespread outbreaks during the 2023/24 season [9]. The Finnish GII.17 strains were part of the globally expanding lineage and provided molecular evidence of their delayed introduction and spread in Finland. This phenomenon is not unique; Finland has experienced delayed emergence of epidemic viral pathogens compared to Central and Southern Europe before [11–13]. The true emergence of GII.17, however, might be undetected, since not all norovirus outbreaks in Finland undergo molecular investigation.

During the COVID-19 pandemic (seasons 2019/20 and 2020/21), no GII.17 norovirus was identified in Finland. Reduced virus transmission can be due to pandemic control measures: social distance, restrictions on dining together and traveling, and more hand washing leading to less outbreak investigations. After the pandemic, detection of GII.17 norovirus resumed. The actual burden of GII.17 norovirus in Finland is probably underestimated since sporadic cases likely represent a chain of person-to-person transmission, especially in settings where outbreak investigations are not routinely conducted. The rise in GII.17 detections during the 2024/25 season suggests a shift in genotype dominance and highlights the dynamic nature of norovirus epidemiology. This may partly be due to the population's lack of exposure to norovirus infections during the pandemic, which could have led to a decline in immunity [14].

Norovirus infections are typically short-lived and self-limiting, and they rarely require hospitalization. As a result, the total number of norovirus cases often remains underreported in official statistics and only a small fraction of patients seek medical care or are recorded [15–17]. During the 2024–2025 season, 42% of FWOR notifications were suspected norovirus outbreaks, yet genotyping was performed in only four cases. This reflects the established practice of conducting genotyping only when exact identification is needed for comparing noroviruses in patients and the suspected source. In such cases, expert consultation is often requested from the Finnish Institute for Health and Welfare (THL), particularly when a food- or waterborne source is suspected.

The recognition of delayed genotype emergence has important public health implications. Although norovirus infections are clinically similar regardless of genotype, the introduction of a novel strain such as GII.17 may lead to larger outbreaks due to a lower population immunity [18–20]. Norovirus is highly contagious and can spread rapidly in institutional and community settings, often before public health interventions can be fully implemented. Thus, awareness of emerging genotypes in other regions may enhance preparedness by heightening surveillance and outbreak detection, and communication with healthcare providers. The public health authorities could also consider integrating international surveillance data into national risk assessments. Still, without targeted interventions or vaccines, the impact of enhanced surveillance and risk assessments may be limited to mitigation rather than prevention. Continued monitoring and international data sharing remain essential tools in mitigating the impact of emerging norovirus strains.

This study has several limitations that should be acknowledged. First, norovirus genotyping in Finland is not routinely performed for all outbreaks or sporadic cases, which may lead to underestimation of the true prevalence and distribution of GII.17. Genotyping is typically reserved for outbreaks with suspected foodborne or waterborne sources, limiting the representativeness of the data. Second, the retrospective nature of the surveillance data may introduce reporting biases, especially in earlier years when genotyping capacity and awareness of GII.17 were lower. Third, the sporadic cases included in this study were selected from diagnostic laboratories, which may not fully capture community transmission dynamics. Additionally, the lack of clinical data and detailed exposure histories for sporadic cases restricts our ability to assess transmission routes and outbreak linkages.

Supplementary Materials: The following supporting information can be downloaded at https://www.mdpi.com/article/10.3390/v17121530/s1. Table S1: Metadata of Norovirus GII.17 and GII.P17 Isolates Collected in Finland (2015–2025).

Author Contributions: H.A.-H. was responsible for the analysis of human samples, wrote the manuscript draft, and is the corresponding author of the article. R.R.-F. was responsible for food- and waterborne outbreak surveillance and contributed to writing of the article. C.S.-K. contributed to writing of the article and acted as the supervisor of the work. All authors have read and agreed to the published version of the manuscript.

Funding: This research received no external funding.

Institutional Review Board Statement: All data used in this study were collected as part of statutory public health surveillance and outbreak investigations. Institutional review board statement is not applicable.

Data Availability Statement: All data generated or analyzed in this study were collected as part of statutory public health surveillance and outbreak investigations. Sequence data have been deposited in GenBank under accession numbers PV973171–PV973223. Additional details are provided in the Supplementary Materials.

Acknowledgments: We would like to express our sincere gratitude to all the municipalities across Finland for their valuable support in outbreak investigations, as well as to the diagnostic laboratories that provided us with human samples. We also acknowledge the collaboration with the Finnish Food Authority, whose contributions were essential to the success of this work.

Conflicts of Interest: We declare no conflicts of interest.

References

1. Platts-Mills, J.A.; Taniuchi, M.; Uddin, M.J.; Sobuz, S.U.; Mahfuz, M.; Gaffar, S.M.A.; Mondal, D.; Hossain, M.I.; Islam, M.M.; Ahmed, A.M.S.; et al. Association between enteropathogens and malnutrition in children aged 6–23 mo in Bangladesh: A case-control study1, 2, 3. *Am. J. Clin. Nutr.* **2017**, *105*, 1132–1138. [CrossRef] [PubMed]
2. Finnish Legislation. Available online: https://www.finlex.fi/fi/lainsaadanto/2011/1365 (accessed on 18 November 2025).
3. Vinjé, J.; Hamidjaja, R.A.; Sobsey, M.D. Development and application of a capsid VP1 (region D) based reverse transcription PCR assay for genotyping of genogroup I and II noroviruses. *J. Virol. Methods* **2004**, *116*, 109–117. [CrossRef] [PubMed]
4. Norovirus Typing Tool Version 2.0. Available online: https://mpf.rivm.nl/mpf/norovirus/typingtool/ (accessed on 18 November 2025).
5. Lindesmith, L.C.; Kocher, J.F.; Donaldson, E.F.; Debbink, K.; Mallory, M.L.; Swann, E.W.; Brewer-Jensen, P.D.; Baric, R.S. Emergence of Novel Human Norovirus GII.17 Strains Correlates with Changes in Blockade Antibody Epitopes. *J. Infect. Dis.* **2017**, *216*, 1227–1234. [CrossRef] [PubMed] [PubMed Central]
6. Zuo, Y.; Xue, L.; Gao, J.; Liao, Y.; Liang, Y.; Jiang, Y.; Cai, W.; Qin, Z.; Yang, J.; Zhang, J.; et al. Evolutionary Mechanism of Immunological Cross-Reactivity Between Different GII.17 Variants. *Front. Microbiol.* **2021**, *12*, 653719. [CrossRef] [PubMed] [PubMed Central]
7. Chhabra, P.; Wong, S.; Niendorf, S.; Lederer, I.; Vennema, H.; Faber, M.; Nisavanh, A.; Jacobsen, S.; Williams, R.; Colgan, A.; et al. Increased circulation of GII.17 noroviruses, six European countries and the United States, 2023 to 2024. *Eurosurveillance* **2024**, *29*, 2400625. [CrossRef] [PubMed] [PubMed Central]
8. Kearse, M.; Moir, R.; Wilson, A.; Stones-Havas, S.; Cheung, M.; Sturrock, S.; Buxton, S.; Cooper, A.; Markowitz, S.; Duran, C.; et al. Geneious Basic: An integrated and extendable desktop software platform for the organization and analysis of sequence data. *Bioinformatics* **2012**, *28*, 1647–1649. [CrossRef] [PubMed] [PubMed Central]
9. Kumar, S.; Stecher, G.; Suleski, M.; Sanderford, M.; Sharma, S.; Tamura, K. MEGA12: Molecular Evolutionary Genetic Analysis Version 12 for Adaptive and Green Computing. *Mol. Biol. Evol.* **2024**, *41*, msae263. [CrossRef] [PubMed] [PubMed Central]
10. Tamura, K.; Nei, M. Estimation of the number of nucleotide substitutions in the control region of mitochondrial DNA in humans and chimpanzees. *Mol. Biol. Evol.* **1993**, *10*, 512–526. [CrossRef] [PubMed]

11. Polkowska, A.; Rönnqvist, M.; Lepistö, O.; Roivainen, M.; Maunula, L.; Huusko, S.; Toikkanen, S.; Rimhanen-Finne, R. Outbreak of gastroenteritis caused by norovirus GII.4 Sydney variant after a wedding reception at a resort/activity centre, Finland, August 2012. *Epidemiol. Infect.* **2014**, *142*, 1877–1883. [CrossRef] [PubMed] [PubMed Central]
12. Summa, M.; Tuutti, E.; Al-Hello, H.; Huttunen, L.M.; Rimhanen-Finne, R. Norovirus GII.17 Caused Five Outbreaks Linked to Frozen Domestic Bilberries in Finland, 2019. *Food Environ. Virol.* **2024**, *16*, 180–187. [CrossRef] [PubMed]
13. Lappe, B.L.; Wikswo, M.E.; Kambhampati, A.K.; Mirza, S.A.; Tate, J.E.; Kraay, A.N.M.; Lopman, B.A. Predicting norovirus and rotavirus resurgence in the United States following the COVID-19 pandemic: A mathematical modelling study. *BMC Infect. Dis.* **2023**, *23*, 254. [CrossRef] [PubMed] [PubMed Central]
14. Carlson, K.B.; Dilley, A.; O'Grady, T.; Johnson, J.A.; Lopman, B.; Viscidi, E. A narrative review of norovirus epidemiology, biology, and challenges to vaccine development. *NPJ Vaccines* **2024**, *9*, 94. [CrossRef] [PubMed] [PubMed Central]
15. Zhu, M.; Huang, Z.; Liu, T.; Wu, C.; Shang, Z.; Zhang, L. Global burden and trends of norovirus-associated diseases from 1990 to 2021 an observational trend study. *Front. Public Health* **2025**, *12*, 1483149. [CrossRef] [PubMed] [PubMed Central]
16. Robilotti, E.; Deresinski, S.; Pinsky, B.A. Norovirus. *Clin. Microbiol. Rev.* **2015**, *28*, 134–164. [CrossRef] [PubMed] [PubMed Central]
17. Rha, B.; Burrer, S.; Park, S.; Trivedi, T.; Parashar, U.D.; Lopman, B.A. Emergency department visit data for rapid detection and monitoring of norovirus activity, United States. *Emerg. Infect. Dis.* **2013**, *19*, 1214–1221. [CrossRef] [PubMed] [PubMed Central]
18. Barclay, L.; Vinjé, J. Increasing Predominance of Norovirus GII.17 over GII.4, United States, 2022–2025. *Emerg. Infect. Dis.* **2025**, *31*, 1471–1473. [CrossRef] [PubMed] [PubMed Central]
19. van Beek, J.; de Graaf, M.; Al-Hello, H.; Allen, D.J.; Ambert-Balay, K.; Botteldoorn, N.; Brytting, M.; Buesa, J.; Cabrerizo, M.; Chan, M.; et al. Molecular surveillance of norovirus, 2005–2016: An epidemiological analysis of data collected from the NoroNet network. *Lancet Infect. Dis.* **2018**, *18*, 545–553. [CrossRef] [PubMed]
20. Lopman, B.; Vennema, H.; Kohli, E.; Pothier, P.; Sanchez, A.; Negredo, A.; Buesa, J.; Schreier, E.; Reacher, M.; Brown, D.; et al. Increase in viral gastroenteritis outbreaks in Europe and epidemic spread of new norovirus variant. *Lancet* **2004**, *363*, 682–688. [CrossRef] [PubMed]

viruses

MDPI

Article

Significant Association Between Increased Abundance of Selected Bacterial Lipopolysaccharides and Norovirus Diarrhea Among South African Infants

Lerato P. Kgosana, Mapaseka L. Seheri and Cliff A. Magwira *

Diarrheal Pathogens Research Unit (DPRU), Department of Medical Virology, Sefako Makgatho Health Sciences University, Pretoria 0208, South Africa; lerato.kgosana@smu.ac.za (L.P.K.); mapaseka.seheri@smu.ac.za (M.L.S.)

* Correspondence: cmagwira@gmail.com or cliff.magwira@smu.ac.za; Tel.: +27-(012)-521-3036

Abstract: Bacterial lipopolysaccharides (LPS) have been shown to promote enteric viral infections. This study assessed whether possessing elevated levels of LPS was associated with norovirus infection. Fecal samples from diarrheic norovirus-positive (DNP) (n = 26), non-diarrheal norovirus-negative (NDNN) (n = 26), asymptomatic norovirus-positive (ANP) (n = 15), and diarrheic norovirus-negative (DNN) (n =15) infants were assayed for selected bacterial LPS by quantitative PCR. The mean levels of selected LPS gene targets were significantly high in DNP infants (6.17 ± 2.14 CFU/g) versus NDNN infants (4.13 ± 2.25 CFU/g), $p = 0.003$. So too was the abundance between DNP and DNN infants ($p = 0.0023$). The levels of selected LPS gene targets were high regardless of whether the infection was symptomatic or asymptomatic, $p = 0.3808$. The average expression of genes coding for selected LPS and their signalling molecule, Toll-like receptor 4 (TLR4), increased 7- and 2.5-fold, respectively, in DNP versus NDNN children. Infants possessing elevated levels of selected LPS-rich bacteria were 1.51 times more likely to develop norovirus diarrhea (95% CI: 1.14–2.01, $p = 0.004$). In conclusion, norovirus infection was associated with abundance of selected bacterial LPS, suggesting a possible role of bacterial LPS in norovirus infection.

Keywords: bacterial lipopolysaccharide; TLR4; norovirus diarrhea; abundance; gene expression

1. Introduction

Norovirus is one of the leading causes of acute viral gastroenteritis (AGE) worldwide, accounting for over 200,000 deaths and 685 million infections in children under the age of 5 [1]. Several host innate factors have been associated with an individual's susceptibility to norovirus infection [2]. Recent studies have also indicated the involvement of commensal bacteria in successful norovirus infections. For instance, norovirus was unable to infect mice treated with antibiotics compared to their untreated counterpart [3]. Several hypotheses that explain how gut bacteria influence enteric viral infection exist, including the effects of bacterial lipopolysaccharides [4]. Lipopolysaccharides (LPS), expressed by mostly Gram-negative bacteria, have been shown to promote enteric viral infections [4]. Binding of the viral particle to bacterial LPS increases its thermostability and resistance to inactivation from chemicals [4]. This subsequently enhances the chance for the virus to infect the target cells, possibly by affording the virus time to reach its target cells. Bacterial LPS also facilitate the attachment of the viral particles to the target cells as the binding of enteric viruses, such as poliovirus to specific receptors, was reported to improve in the presence of bacterial LPS, suggesting that the LPS is directly involved in the attachment of enteric viruses to target cells [4].

The viral binding is not limited to bacterial LPS as studies have shown that the viruses also bind to other bacterial components including N-acetylglucosamine-containing surface polysaccharides that are longer than six monosaccharides [5]. N-acelylglucosamine is a main component of bacterial cell wall peptidoglycan that is made up of a sugar backbone consisting of alternating residues of β-(1,4) linked N-acetylglucosamine and N-acetylmuramic acid [6]. When combined with uridine diphosphate (UDP), N-acetylglucosamine is also a precursor for the synthesis of the lipid A of LPS, which is a major part of the outer membrane of Gram-negative bacteria [7].

Bacterial LPS is a tripartite structure consisting of the lipid A that docks the LPS to the outer membrane; core oligosaccharide, which maintain the integrity of the outer membrane; and O antigen polysaccharide or O antigen, which is connected to the core and made up of a polymer of repetitive oligosaccharide units exposed to and interacting with the external environment [8]. While the genes that code for common polysaccharide are conserved, there is little homology in different set of genes responsible for the biosynthesis of the O-specific antigen in different bacteria, making it impossible to target a single gene to quantify the O antigen of the LPS.

Several intestinal Gram-negative bacteria such as *Serratia marcescens*, *Klebsiella pneumoniae*, *Pseudomonas aeruguinosa*, and others are reported to be rich in LPS and other N acetylglucosamine-containing surface polysaccharides [9,10]. However, despite their significance, little is known about the role of the abundance of LPS-rich bacteria and other N acetylglucosamine-containing surface polysaccharides in pediatric norovirus infection. Here, we report that harbouring increased levels of LPS-rich bacteria and other N acetylglucosamine-containing surface polysaccharides can be a risk factor for pediatric norovirus diarrhea.

2. Methods

2.1. Study Design, Population, and Sampling

This is a case–control study that used stool samples collected from infants attending Oukasie Healthcare Clinic, north of Pretoria for a routine vaccination programme and diarrhea between 2018 and 2020. Diarrhea was defined as having episodes of at least three loose, watery stools within 24 h, along with at least one of the following symptoms: nausea, vomiting, abdominal pain, or high fever [11]. Stool samples were collected from infants of similar age (3.5 and 9 months) after written and informed consent from the parents. The study cases were limited to these specific months as the study controls were enrolled at a vaccination clinic for rotavirus immunization at 3.5 and 9.0 months of age. Study participants were divided into four groups: diarrheic norovirus-positive (DNP), asymptomatic norovirus-positive (ANP), non-diarrheic norovirus-negative (NDNN), and diarrheic norovirus-negative infants (DNN). Infants on antibiotic therapy or treated with antibiotics 4 weeks prior to recruitment were excluded from the study. Ethical clearance was approved by the Sefako Makgatho Health Sciences University Research and Ethics Committee, SMUREC/M199/2020: PG.

Stool samples were collected from the infants' diapers into sterile plastic bottles. Watery stool samples were collected by squeezing the soiled part of the diaper into the bottle and immediately freezing at −20 °C and transporting to the laboratory within 30 min in cooler boxes packed with ice blocks.

2.2. Stool Viral RNA and Bacterial Genomic DNA Extraction

Viral RNA was extracted from 10% (*w*/*v*) stool suspension using a Viral RNA Mini Extraction Kit (Qiagen, Hilden, Germany) following the manufacturer's instructions with minor modifications [12]. Viral RNA was eluted in 50 µL buffer and stored at −20 °C for short-term storage and −80 °C for long-term storage. DNA was extracted from stool samples using QIAamp Fast DNA Stool Mini Kit (Qiagen, Hilden, Germany) following the manufacturer's guidelines. A total of 150 µL of fecal DNA was eluted and stored at −80 °C.

2.3. Detection of Norovirus in Stool Samples

Stool viral RNA was assayed for the presence of norovirus by reverse transcriptase polymerase chain reaction (RT-qPCR) using Allplex GI-Virus Assay kit (Seegene, Seoul, Republic of Korea) as recommended by the manufacturer. RT-qPCR assay was performed in a Bio-Rad CFX96 Real-Time System (Bio-Rad Laboratories, Hercules, CA, USA) using a 96-well plate (Nunc, Roskilde, Denmark) and the results were analyzed in a Seegene Viewer (Seegene, Seoul, Republic of Korea). A cycle threshold (Ct) value of 40 or below was considered as positive for norovirus [13].

2.4. Quantitative PCR Assay for Detection of Selected LPS-Rich Bacteria and Sequencing

Bacterial N-acetylglucosamine and selected LPS-rich bacteria were assayed in the stool DNA samples by qPCR using bacterial N-acetylglucosamine and LPS species-specific primers and probes (this study) (Table 1) that targeted the genes coding for synthesis of bacterial N-acetylglucosamine (GlmU) and LPS of *K. pneumonia* (*Waa*E), *S. marcescens* (*kdt*X), and *P. aeruginosa* (*Waa*L).

Table 1. Primers and probes used in this study.

Species/Compound	Name and Sequences	Gene	Ref
P. aeruginosa	WaaLF-CCAGATCAGCGAGCATCCAT WaaLR-CGAAAAGCACACCCAGTTCG WaaLP-Texas red-CGGCTACGATCATCCGAT- BHQ-2	*Waa*L	This study
S. marcescens	WaaF-TCGACGGTAAACAGGGGTTG WaaR-TCACTTCTCTGAGTAGTTGCGG WaaP-Hex-TAGCGGTGGTCAACGCGCAATATA-BHQ-1	*kdt*X	This study
K. pneumoniae	WaaEF-TCGTTATAGCGGTAACGGGC WaaER-TCGCCCGCCGTAACTATTTT WaaEP-Hex-ATACCAACCGCTGTGGCGCATAAA-BHQ-1	*Waa*E	This study
N-acetylglucosamine	GlmU-F-GTGATGTAGTATTCGCCCTGAG GlmU-R-AAGATGCCACCGACGAGCAG GlmU-P FAM-TTGTTGGTCAGCTTCGCCAG-BHQ-1	*Glm*U	This study
Toll-like receptor 4	TLR4 F-GATTGCTCAGACCTGGCAGTT TLR4 R-GTCCTCCCACTCCAGGTAAGT	TLR4	This study

Quantitative PCR amplification was performed in a Bio-Rad CFX96 Real-Time System (Bio-Rad Laboratories, Hercules, CA, USA) using 8-tube PCR strips (Bio-Rad Laboratories, Watford, UK). The 20 µL reaction mix was made up of 2X Luna Universal qPCR Master Mix (New England BioLabs, Ipswich, MA, USA), 0.25 µM each of the probe, forward and reverse primer, 5 µL bacterial DNA, and nucleic free water. The qPCR assay was performed under the following conditions: initial denaturation at 95 °C for 5 min, 45 cycles of 95 °C for 15 s, and 60 °C for 30 s. Conventional PCR products obtained by amplification of selected gene targets using species specific primers (Table 1) were sanger-sequenced (Inqaba Biotech, Pretoria, South Africa) to confirm their identity.

2.5. Bacterial Quantification Standards

The standard curves used to quantify the selected LPS-rich bacteria were prepared from genomic DNA extracted from *K. pneumoniae* (ATCC: BAA-2146), *S. marcescens* (ATCC: 43862), and *P. aeruginosa* (ATCC: 27853). In summary, for each bacterial strain used, cultures were inoculated in Luria–Bertani broth (Gibco, Dublin, Ireland) until the strains were in the logarithmic growth phase. Tenfold serial dilutions were prepared and plated in triplicate on nutrient agar plates to enumerate the bacterial colony-forming units (CFU). The remainder of each serial dilution was used to extract the DNA. The extracted DNA was used to generate standard curves by plotting the qPCR Ct value of each dilution against the corresponding CFU.

2.6. Bacterial mRNA Extraction and cDNA Synthesis

Bacterial mRNA was extracted from 10% stool (*w*/*v*) suspension using NucleoSpin Mini RNA kit (Machinery Nagel, Duran, Germany) following the manufacturer's instructions. Complementary DNA (cDNA) was synthesized using Tetro cDNA Synthesis kit (Bioline Inc., Tauton, MA, USA). A 20 µL reaction mix consisted of 1 µL random hexamers, 1 µL of 10 mM dNTPs mix, 4 µL of 5x RT Buffer, 1 µL RiboSafe RNase Inhibitor, 200 u of reverse transcriptase, 7 µL RNase-free water, and 5 µL RNA template. The reverse transcriptase reaction was performed under the following conditions: 25 °C for 10 min, followed by 45 °C for 30 min, and 85 °C for 5 min; the reaction was immediately chilled on ice and stored at −20 °C until further use.

2.7. LPS and TLR4 Gene Expression

The expression of the selected LPS and TLR4 genes in stool mRNA samples was determined by real-time PCR using HOT FIREPol® EvaGreen® qPCR Mix Plus (ROX) (Solis BioDyne, Tartu, Estonia) and primers listed in Table 1 as recommended by the manufacturer with minor modifications. Briefly, the 20 µL reaction mixture consisted of 1X HOT FIREPol® EvaGreen®qPCR Mix Plus, 400 nM of both forward and reverse primers, 5 µL of the cDNA template and the remainder was made PCR grade water. The qPCR was performed in Bio-Rad CFX96 Real-Time System (Bio-Rad Laboratories, Hercules, CA, USA) under the following conditions: 95 °C for 5 min and 45 cycles of 95 °C for 10 s and 60 °C for 15 s. A melting curve was included in the analysis to differentiate between true positives and primer dimers. Values of the LPS and TLR4 gene expressions were normalized against the housekeeping GAPDH and calculated as previously described [14]. The difference in gene expression was presented as fold change.

2.8. Statistical Analysis

Differences in demographics between the diarrhea norovirus-positive and non-diarrhea norovirus-negative infants were determined by the χ^2 test. The bacterial CFU/g counts were converted to a logarithmic form while descriptive statistics were presented in terms of mean and standard deviation and displayed as box plots using Graphpad Prism 9.2.0 (GraphPad Software, San Diego, CA, USA). A Mann–Whitney U test was used to determine differences in levels of selected LPS-rich bacteria between the study groups. Bacterial CFU/g were used as a continuous variable to test the association between bacterial levels of selected LPS-rich bacteria and norovirus diarrhea using logistical regression. Multiple logistical regression analysis was also used to assess the contribution of potential confounding factors in predicting levels of the selected LPS-rich bacteria and bacteria N-acetylglucosamine. The difference in fold expression of the selected genes was presented as mean and standard deviation and was analyzed with a parametric unpaired *t*-test with

Welch's correction. The normality in the distribution of the data was determined with the Kolmogorov–Smirnov test. A *p*-value less than or equal to 0.05 was considered significant.

3. Results

3.1. Demographics and Other Characteristics

No significant differences were observed in demographics and other characteristics between diarrheic norovirus-positive and non-diarrheic norovirus-negative groups (Table 2). Similarly, there were no significant differences in the demographics between asymptomatic norovirus-positive and diarrheic norovirus-negative infants.

Table 2. Demographics and other baseline characteristics between diarrheic norovirus-positive (DNP) and non-diarrheic norovirus-negative (NNDN) infants.

Characteristics		**DNP n (%)**	**NDNN n (%)**	***p* Value**
Gender	Female	12 (46)	10 (39)	0.5745
	Male	14 (54)	16 (61)	
Age	3.5 months	14 (54)	11 (42)	0.4050
	9 months	12 (46)	15 (58)	
Mode of delivery	Natural birth	20 (77)	17 (65)	0.3584
	Caesarean	6 (23)	9 (35)	
Feeding type	Breast milk	25 (96)	23 (88)	0.2979
	Formula	1 (04)	3 (12)	

3.2. Abundance of Selected LPS-Rich Bacteria and N-Acetylglucosamine in Diarrheic Norovirus-Positive and Non-Diarrheic Norovirus-Negative Infants

A total of 178 diarrheic infants were enrolled into the study and assayed for norovirus infection. Of the 178 infants, 26 were positive for norovirus and were, together with 26 non-diarrheic norovirus-negative from a cohort attending an immunization programme, 15 asymptomatic norovirus-positive and 15 diarrheic norovirus-negative infants, used to evaluate differences in levels of bacterial N-acetylglucosamine and selected LPS-rich bacteria. The results, expressed as a log colony-forming unit per gram (CFU/g), are shown in Figures 1–3. The average levels of selected LPS gene targets were significantly high in DNP infants (6.17 ± 2.14 CFU/g) compared to their NDNN counterparts (4.13 ± 2.25 CFU/g), p = 0.003 (Figure 1a). Similarly, DNP infants harboured significantly higher levels of N-acetylglucosamine (7.33 ± 1.11 CFU/g) than NDNN infants (5.484 ± 2.18), p = 0.0205 (Figure 3a). Individually, DNP infants possessed significantly high levels of *S. marcescens* (8.47 ± 4.04 CFU/g) compared to their non-diarrheic norovirus-negative peers (5.52 ± 4.24 CFU/g), p = 0.0074 (Figure 2e). So too were the levels of *K. pneumoniae* in DNP infants (5.39 ± 2.28 CFU/g) versus NDNN infants (3.28 ± 1.86 CFU/g), p = 0.0264 (Figure 2a). There was no significant difference in levels of *P. aeruginosa* between the two study groups (p = 0.1629) (Figure 2i).

When compared to infants with diarrhea due other enteric pathogens, the mean abundance of all selected LPS gene targets were significantly high in DNP infants (6.17 ± 2.14 CFU/g) compared to DNN infants (3.67 ± 2.05 CFU/g), p = 0.0023 (Figure 1c). Similarly, DNP infants contained significantly higher levels of N-acetylglucosamine (7.33 ± 1.11 CFU/g) than DNN infants (5.72 ± 2.44 CFU/g), p = 0.0399 (Figure 3c). However, there was no difference in the mean abundance of all selected LPS gene targets as well as N-acetylglucosamine in DNP and their asymptomatic (ANP) counterparts, p = 0.3480 and 0.1262, respectively (Figures 1b and 2b). Individually, significantly higher levels of *S. marcescens* and *K pneumoniae* were observed in DNP infants (8.47 ± 4.04 CFU/g and 5.39 ± 2.28 CFU/g, respectively) compared to their DNN counterparts (4.19 ± 2.75 CFU/g and 3.16 ± 2.09 CFU/g), p = 0.0007 and 0.0342, respectively (Figure 2g,c). Except for *S. marcescens* (p = 0.0330) (Figure 2f), there were no significant differences between the levels of N-acetylglucosamine and *K pneumoniae* in DNP and ANP infants, p = 0.1262 and 0.9058, respectively (Figures 1b and 2b).

When abundance was stratified according to age, 3.5 and 9 month-old DNP infants contained significantly higher levels of all selected LPS-rich bacteria (5.92 ± 2.56 CFU/g) and (6.69 ± 2.11 CFU/g), respectively, compared to their NDNN counterparts (3.73 ± 2.76 CFU/g) and (4.16 ± 3.02 CFU/g), p = 0.0331 and 0.0210, respectively (Figure 1d,e). The levels of N-acetylglucosamine were only significantly higher in 9-month-old DNP (6.69 ± 2.34 CFU/g) than 9-month-old NDNN infants (6.02 ± 2.13 CFU/g), p = 0.0335 (Figure 3d). So too was the level of *S. marcescens* in 9-month-old DNP infants (8.36 ± 3.42 CFU/g) compared to non-diarrheic norovirus-negative peers and (4.71 ± 3.08 CFU/g), p = 0.0140 (Figure 2h). On the other hand, 3.5-months-old diarrheic norovirus-positive infants harboured significantly higher levels of *K. pneumoniae* (4.34 ± 2.65 CFU/g) than non-diarrheic norovirus-negative infants (2.08 ± 1.57 CFU/g), p = 0.0169 (Figure 2d).

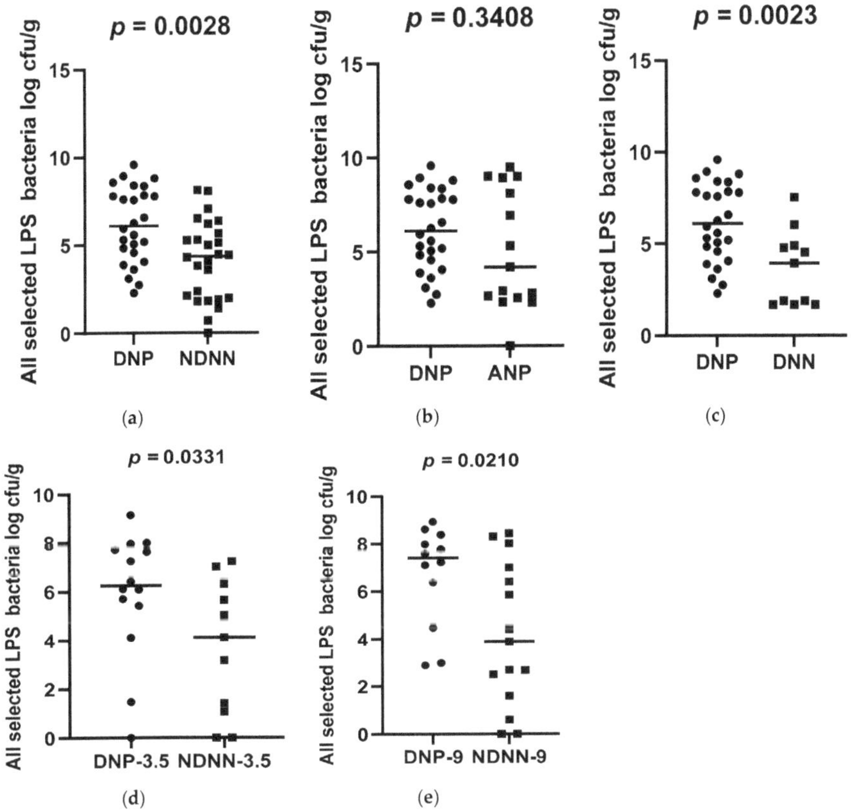

Figure 1. Average abundance of all selected LPS-rich bacteria in (**a**) DNP vs. NDNN (**b**) DNP vs. ANP (**c**) DNP vs. DNN (**d**) DNP vs. NDNN at 3.5 months of age, (**e**) DNP vs. NDNN at 9 months of age. — denotes the mean.

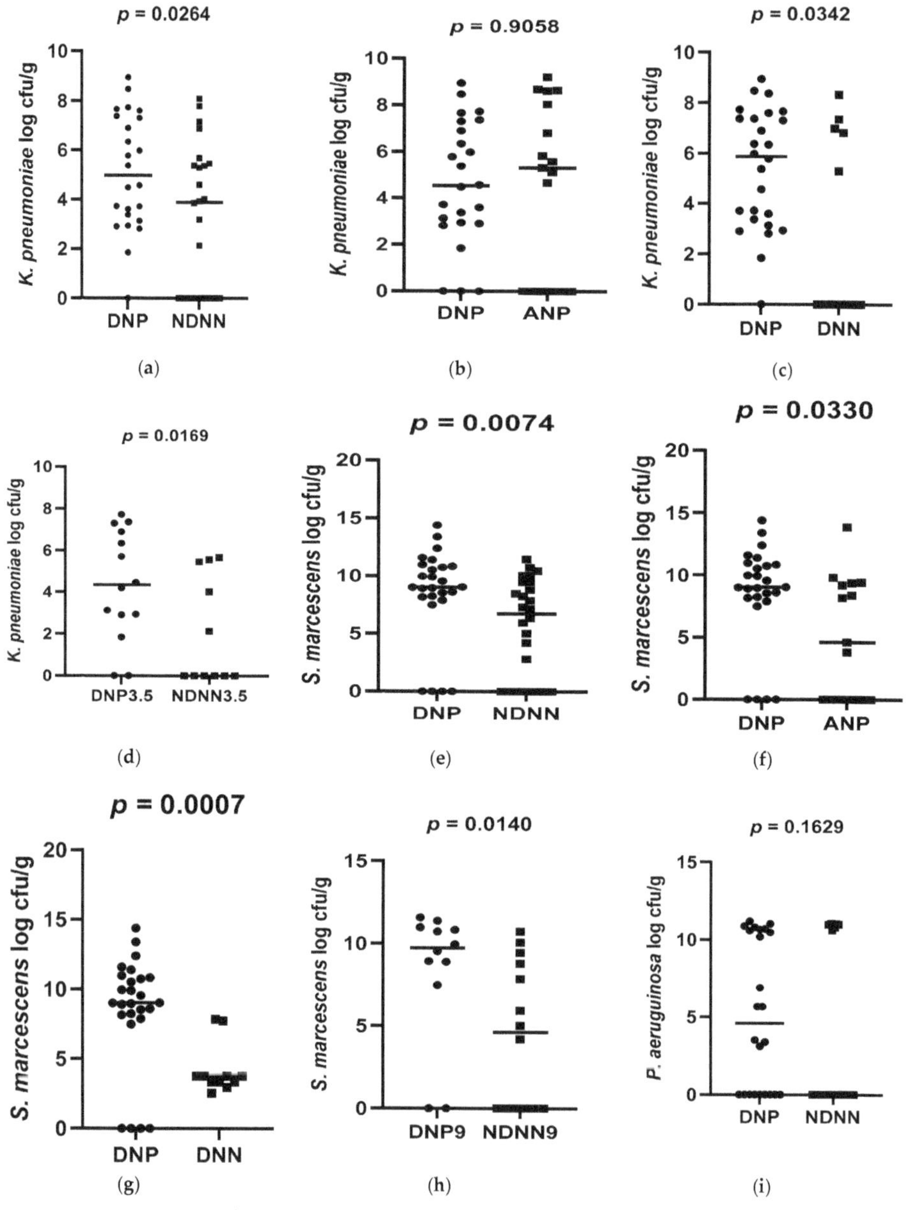

Figure 2. Abundance of each of the selected LPS-rich bacteria in (**a**) DNP vs. NDNN (*K. pneumonia*), (**b**) DNP vs. ANP (*K. pneumonia*), (**c**) DNP vs. DNN (*K. pneumonia*), (**d**) DNP vs. NDNN (*K. pneumonia*) at 3.5 months old (**e**) DNP vs. NDNN (*S. marcescens*), (**f**) DNP vs. ANP (*S. marcescens*), (**g**) DNP vs. DNN (*S. marcescens*), (**h**) DNP9 vs. NDNN9 (*S. marcescens*), (**i**) DNP vs. NDNN (*P. aeruginosa*).

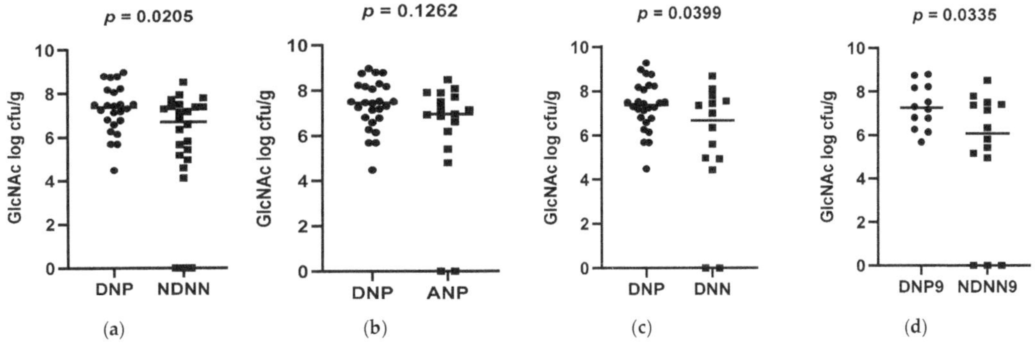

Figure 3. Abundance of N-acetylglucosamine in all selected bacteria (**a**) DNP vs. NDNN (**b**) DNP vs. ANP (**c**) DNP vs. DNN (**d**) DNP vs. NDNN at 9 months of age.

3.3. Expression of the Select LPS, N-Acetylglucosamine and TLR4 in Stool mRNA Samples

The expression levels of the bacterial LPS genes (*Waa*E for *K. pneumoniae*, and *kdtX* for *S. marcescens* as well as *Glm*U for bacterial N-acetylglucosamine) were compared between DNP and NDNN samples. There was a 7-fold increase in average expression of all selected LPS genes in DNP infants compared to their NDNN counterparts (Figure 4a). Individually, there was a 4.7- and 17-fold increase in average expression of *Waa*E and *KdtX* genes, respectively, in DNP infants compared to NDNN infants (Figure 4b,c). On the other hand, the average expression of GlmU decreased 10-fold in DNP compared to their NDNN counterparts (Figure 4d). The expression of TLR4 in fecal samples was consistent with the abundance of the LPS as it increased 2.5-fold in DRP children compared to NDRN children (Figure 4e).

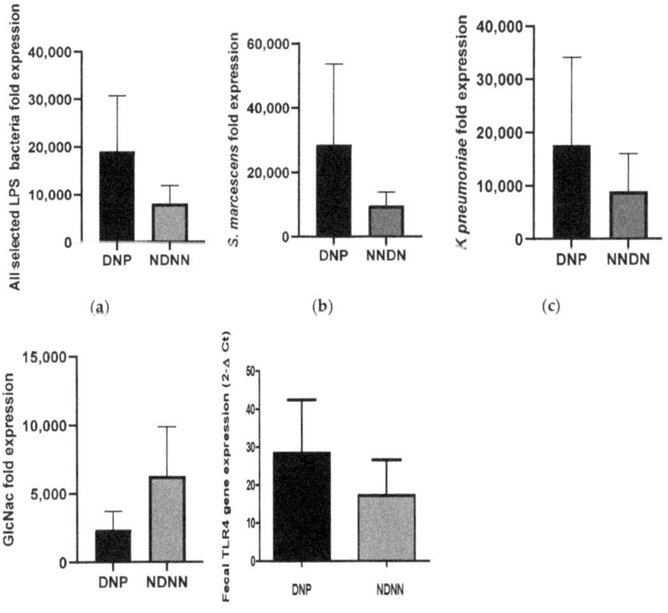

Figure 4. Expression of LPS genes of selected LPS-rich bacteria, N-acetylglucosamine and TLR4 between DNP and NDNN study groups: (**a**) mean of all selected LPS genes, (**b**) *S. marcescens*, (**c**) *K. pneumoniae*, (**d**) N-acetylglucosamine, and (**e**) TLR4.

3.4. Association Between the Abundance of Bacterial LPS and Norovirus Diarrhea

The average levels of selected LPS-rich bacteria in stool samples of DNP and NDNN were used as a continuous variable to evaluate its association with norovirus diarrhea. Infants harbouring increased levels of bacterial LPS were more likely to have norovirus diarrhea compared to those with low levels of the compound (odds ratio [OR] = 1.51, 95% confidence interval [CI] = 1.14–2.01, $p = 0.033$). Other potential confounding factors such as sex, mode of delivery, and feeding type did not contribute in predicting the levels of selected LPS gene target in the infants (OR = 0.899, 95% CI: 0.6832–1.1829, $p = 0.447$; OR = 1.037, 95% CI: 0.7638–1.4092, $p = 0.814$; and OR = 0.8726, 95% CI: 0.4966–1.5333, $p = 0.637$, respectively.

4. Discussion

The study found significantly higher levels of bacterial N-acetylglucosamine and selected LPS-rich bacteria in DNP children compared to their NDNN counterparts. Lack of homology between LPS genes in different bacteria rendered designing of primers to target all bacterial LPS in stool samples impossible; as such the study used the three selected bacteria as representative of LPS-rich bacteria. Nevertheless, the findings suggest that elevated levels of bacterial LPS may play a role in norovirus infection and diarrhea. In fact, logistical regression analysis of bacterial counts and norovirus diarrhea indicated an association between the level of fecal bacterial LPS and the disease. Elevated levels of LPS-rich bacteria mean more noroviruses will be able to bind to LPS, survive harsh intestinal conditions and become facilitated to attach and infect the target cells (affording the virus more time to reach its target) [4,5] and cause diarrhea. The mechanism through which bacterial LPS stabilizes norovirus is not fully explained but it is thought the negative charge of the LPS (due to phosphate group) interacts with the charged region of norovirus capsid, thereby preventing viral conformational change essential for viral inactivation and providing viral stability. Nevertheless, our findings are the first to show association between abundance of LPS and norovirus infection. However, a recent similar study observed that the accumulation of LPS secreted by enriched Gram-negative bacteria was a risk factor for rotavirus colonization in young adults [15].

The abundance of LPS-rich bacteria was assayed using qPCR, which gives an estimate of genome copy numbers but not viable counts of the bacteria. To estimate the level of viable bacteria, the study assayed the expression of gene coding for LPS genes of the selected bacteria between DNP and NDNN infants. Consistent with the abundance of the bacterial LPS gene targets, the average expression of all selected LPS genes were 7-fold higher in DNP than in NDNN. In contrast, the expression of the gene coding for N-acetylglucosamine was much less in DNP infants compared to NDNN infants, suggesting that N-acetylglucosamine from non-viable cells constituted much of total bacterial N-acetylglucosamine assayed. Nonetheless, studies have shown that enhancement of enteric viral infectivity does not require viable bacteria as lipopolysaccharides alone have been shown to directly bind to enteric viruses and promote infection [4].

The mean levels of selected LPS gene targets were high regardless of whether the infection was symptomatic or asymptomatic. It is not known whether the asymptomatic norovirus-positive infants were truly asymptomatic as human studies have indicated [16] or were merely recovering from norovirus diarrhea at the time of sampling that may indicate the continuing fecal norovirus shedding from past infection. Nevertheless, the observation suggests that elevated levels of bacterial LPS could be a susceptibility factor for both norovirus diarrhea and asymptomatic norovirus infection.

The expression of TLR4 gene in the current study corresponded with abundance or expression of selected bacterial LPS. This is consistent with studies in mice, which have shown that LPS activation of the TLR4 gene proceeds in a dose-dependent manner [17]. Immune signalling of LPS occurs via TLR4 and its increase in expression in stool samples of DNP children observed in the current study suggest that LPS may have a role in norovirus infection. The induction of TLR4 can lead to the release of proinflammatory cytokines such as interleukin 6 and 8 (IL-6 and 8) that have been associated with norovirus infections [18]. It is possible that an increase in expression of TLR4 in DRP as the result of higher abundance of LPS resulted in increased levels of IL-6 and IL-8 that created a conducive environment for norovirus infection and diarrhea.

Composition of the gut bacteria can temporarily change due to several physiological conditions including diarrhea. Diarrhea destabilizes the gut environment by increasing bowel movement and fluid secretion that can lead to gut microbiome dysbiosis [19]. The significant differences in abundance of selected bacteria LPS gene targets between DNP and DNN infants observed in the current study suggest that diarrhea could not be the cause of elevated levels of the selected LPS-rich bacteria in DNP infants since both study groups had diarrhea.

When age was stratified, the study observed that differences in levels of fecal bacterial N-acetylglucosamine and LPS-rich *S. marcescens* in diarrheic norovirus-positive and non-diarrheic norovirus-negative infants were notable in 9-month-old infants compared to their 3.5-month old counterparts. The levels of *K. pneumoniae*, on the other hand, were more significant in 3.5-month-old infants than 9-month-olds. During the first two years of life, the composition of gut bacteria is dynamic [19], and the observation in the current study suggests that at any particular time, elevated levels of these LPS-rich bacteria or bacterial N-acetylglucosamine could predispose infants to norovirus diarrhea.

The study also observed that sex, mode of delivery, and feeding type did not contribute significantly in predicting the levels of bacterial N-acetylglucosamine and selected LPS-rich bacteria among the study infants. There have been conflicting reports about differences in gut bacterial abundance between males and females, with some suggesting there is a difference between the two [20–23], while others suggest none [24]. The observation in the current study is in agreement with the latter and could be one of the reasons why both genders are equally affected by norovirus [22]. As the levels and diversity of intestinal bacteria during the first year of life is dynamic and unsteady [19], it is not surprising that the abundance of bacterial N-acetylglucosamine and the selected LPS-rich bacteria in infants' fecal samples could be not predicted according the three confounding factors.

The study had limitations, the first being the small number of samples used to evaluate the differences in levels of bacterial N-acetylglucosamine and selected LPS-rich bacteria between the two study groups. Further studies, with a large sample size, are warranted to validate the current study observations. Secondly, the study population comprised only black South African infants, and since there are reported differences in diversity and composition of bacterial species and strains among different ethnic populations, it would be intriguing to find out the levels of bacterial N-acetylglucosamine and selected LPS-rich bacteria in other ethnic or racial groups. Thirdly, due to little homology of gene coding for the synthesis of LPS, quantification of LPS was only performed for selected LPS-rich bacteria and future studies involving quantification of overall bacterial LPS, possibly through chromatography, is required. Lastly, stool samples are not true indicators of the abundance of bacteria in the intestines where norovirus are suspected to primarily infect. However, they are frequently used as proxies for gut bacteria as they can be collected naturally and non-invasively.

In summary, the study has shown that diarrheic norovirus-positive infants contained significantly high levels of bacterial N-acetylglucosamine and selected LPS-rich bacteria compared to their non-diarrheic norovirus-negative counters. In addition, the expression of LPS signalling molecules increased 2.5-fold in infants with norovirus diarrhea compared to the controls. Infants possessing elevated levels of selected LPS-rich bacteria were more likely to have norovirus diarrhea. The results suggest the possible role of the abundance of bacterial LPS in norovirus infection.

Author Contributions: L.P.K. conducted laboratory investigations and drafted the manuscript. C.A.M. conceptualized the study, supervised, and approved the manuscript, and M.L.S. supervised, and approved the manuscript. All authors have read and agreed to the published version of the manuscript.

Funding: The authors were supported by the National Research Foundation, Grant #138715 (L.P.), Sefako Makgatho Health Sciences University, Grant #134 (C.A.); and South African Medical Research Council (SAMRC) RDA (M.L.).

Institutional Review Board Statement: Ethical clearance for the study was approved by the Sefako Makgatho Health Sciences University Re-search and Ethics Committee, SMUREC/M199/2020: PG.

Informed Consent Statement: Specimen were collected after informed and written consent from parents or guardians of the study infants.

Data Availability Statement: The raw data supporting the conclusions of this article will be made available by the corresponding author on request.

Conflicts of Interest: The authors declare no potential conflicts of interest.

References

1. Shah, M.P.; Hall, A.J. Global Disease Burden of Foodborne Illnesses Associated with Norovirus. In *The Norovirus*; Elsevier: Amsterdam, The Netherlands, 2017; pp. 3–19. [CrossRef]
2. Harrington, P.R.; Vinjé, J.; Moe, C.L.; Baric, R.S. Norovirus Capture with Histo-Blood Group Antigens Reveals Novel Virus-Ligand Interactions. *J. Virol.* **2004**, *78*, 3035–3045. [CrossRef] [PubMed]
3. Jones, M.K.; Watanabe, M.; Zhu, S.; Graves, C.L.; Keyes, L.R.; Grau, K.R.; Gonzalez-Hernandez, M.B.; Iovine, N.M.; Wobus, C.E.; Vinjé, J.; et al. Enteric bacteria promote human and mouse norovirus infection of B cells. *Science* **2014**, *346*, 755–759. [CrossRef]
4. Robinson, C.M.; Jesudhasan, P.R.; Pfeiffer, J.K. Bacterial lipopolysaccharide binding enhances virion stability and promotes en-vironmental fitness of an enteric virus. *Cell Host Microbe* **2014**, *15*, 36–46. [CrossRef]
5. Kuss, S.K.; Best, G.T.; Etheredge, C.A.; Pruijssers, A.J.; Frierson, J.M.; Hooper, L.V.; Dermody, T.S.; Pfeiffer, J.K. Intestinal microbiota promote enteric virus replication and systemic pathogenesis. *Science* **2011**, *334*, 249–252. [CrossRef]
6. Park, J.T.; Uehara, T. How Bacteria Consume Their Own Exoskeletons (Turnover and Recycling of Cell Wall Peptidoglycan). *Microbiol. Mol. Biol. Rev.* **2008**, *72*, 211–227. [CrossRef]
7. Raetz, C.R.H.; Whitfield, C. Lipopolysaccharide endotoxins. *Annu. Rev. Biochem.* **2002**, *71*, 635–700. [CrossRef]
8. Whitfield, C.; Trent, M.S. Biosynthesis and Export of Bacterial Lipopolysaccharides. *Annu. Rev. Biochem.* **2014**, *83*, 99–128. [CrossRef]
9. Bartelt, L.A.; Guerrant, R.L. Antibiotics help control rotavirus infections and enhance antirotaviral immunity: Are you serious? *J. Infect. Dis.* **2014**, *210*, 167–170. [CrossRef]
10. Vatanen, T.; Kostic, A.D.; d'Hennezel, E.; Siljander, H.; Franzosa, E.A.; Yassour, M.; Kolde, R.; Vlamakis, H.; Arthur, T.D.; Hämäläinen, A.-M.; et al. Variation in Microbiome LPS Immunogenicity Contributes to Autoimmunity in Humans. *Cell* **2016**, *165*, 842–853. [CrossRef]
11. A Levine, G.; Walson, J.L.; E Atlas, H.; Lamberti, L.M.; Pavlinac, P.B. Defining Pediatric Diarrhea in Low-Resource Settings. *J. Pediatr. Infect. Dis. Soc.* **2017**, *6*, 289–293. [CrossRef]
12. Magwira, C.A.; Kgosana, L.P.; Esona, M.D.; Seheri, M.L. Low fecal rotavirus vaccine virus shedding is significantly associated with non-secretor histo-blood group antigen phenotype among infants in northern Pretoria, South Africa. *Vaccine* **2020**, *38*, 8260–8263. [CrossRef] [PubMed]
13. Han, J.-H.; Kim, S.-H.; Paik, S.-Y. Evaluation of an Assay Based On Multiple Detection Temperature Technique for Simultaneous Detection of Viral Gastroenteritis-Causing Pathogens. *Jundishapur J. Microbiol.* **2017**, *10*, e43548. [CrossRef]
14. Schmittgen, T.D.; Livak, K.J. Analyzing real-time PCR data by the comparative C_T method. *Nat. Protoc.* **2008**, *3*, 1101–1108. [CrossRef] [PubMed]

15. Wu, Y.; Pei, S.; Wu, J.; Tu, X.; Ren, L.; Ji, Y.; Yao, Y.; Liu, Y. The Abnormal Accumulation of Lipopolysaccharide Secreted by Enriched Gram-Negative Bacteria Increases the Risk of Rotavirus Colonization in Young Adults. *Microorganisms* **2023**, *11*, 2280. [CrossRef]
16. Newman, K.L.; Moe, C.L.; Kirby, A.E.; Flanders, W.D.; Parkos, C.A.; Leon, J.S. Norovirus in symptomatic and asymptomatic individuals: Cytokines and viral shedding. *Clin. Exp. Immunol.* **2016**, *184*, 347–357. [CrossRef]
17. Chen, S.-M.; Lin, C.-P.; Tsai, J.-D.; Chao, Y.-H.; Sheu, J.-N. The Significance of Serum and Fecal Levels of Interleukin-6 and Interleukin-8 in Hospitalized Children with Acute Rotavirus and Norovirus Gastroenteritis. *Pediatr. Neonatol.* **2013**, *55*, 120–126. [CrossRef]
18. Rodrigues, A.; Queiróz, D.B.; Honda, L.; Silva, E.J.R.; Hall, S.H.; Avellar, M.C.W. Activation of Toll-Like Receptor 4 (TLR4) by In Vivo and In Vitro Exposure of Rat Epididymis to Lipopolysaccharide from Escherichia Coli1. *Biol. Reprod.* **2008**, *79*, 1135–1147. [CrossRef]
19. The, H.C.; Le, S.-N.H. Dynamic of the human gut microbiome under infectious diarrhea. *Curr. Opin. Microbiol.* **2022**, *66*, 79–85. [CrossRef]
20. Palmer, C.; Bik, E.M.; DiGiulio, D.B.; Relman, D.A.; Brown, P.O. Development of the Human Infant Intestinal Microbiota. *PLoS Biol.* **2007**, *5*, 1556–1573. [CrossRef]
21. Lay, C.; Rigottier-Gois, L.; Holmstrøm, K.; Rajilic, M.; Vaughan, E.E.; de Vos, W.M.; Collins, M.D.; Thiel, R.; Namsolleck, P.; Blaut, M.; et al. Colonic Microbiota Signatures across Five Northern European Countries. *Appl. Environ. Microbiol.* **2005**, *71*, 4153–4155. [CrossRef]
22. Dominianni, C.; Sinha, R.; Goedert, J.J.; Pei, Z.; Yang, L.; Hayes, R.B.; Ahn, J. Sex, Body Mass Index, and Dietary Fiber Intake Influence the Human Gut Microbiome. *PLoS ONE* **2015**, *10*, e0124599. [CrossRef] [PubMed]
23. Singh, P.; Manning, S.D. Impact of age and sex on the composition and abundance of the intestinal microbiota in individuals with and without enteric infections. *Ann. Epidemiology* **2016**, *26*, 380–385. [CrossRef] [PubMed]
24. Wang, Y.; Hao, L.; Pan, L.; Xue, C.; Liu, Q.; Zhao, X.; Zhu, W. Age, primary symptoms, and genotype characteristics of norovirus outbreaks in Shanghai schools in 2017. *Sci. Rep.* **2018**, *8*, 15238. [CrossRef] [PubMed]

viruses

MDPI

Article

Rotavirus alphagastroenteritidis: Circulating Strains After the Introduction of the Rotavirus Vaccine (Rotarix®) in Luanda Province of Angola

Dikudila G. Vita [1,†], Cristina Santiso-Bellón [2,3,†], Manuel Lemos [1], Zoraima Neto [4], Elsa Fortes-Gabriel [5,6], Miguel Brito [5,7], Cruz S. Sebastião [4,5,8], Jesus Rodriguez-Diaz [2,3], Celso Cunha [9,*] and Claudia Istrate [10,11,*]

1 Faculty of Medicine, Agostinho Neto University, Luanda P.O. Box 116, Angola; dikudilavita@gmail.com (D.G.V.); manuel.lemos90@yahoo.com.br (M.L.)
2 Department of Microbiology, School of Medicine, University of Valencia, Av. Blasco Ibáñez 15, 46010 Valencia, Spain; cristina.santiso@uv.es (C.S.-B.); jesus.rodriguez@uv.es (J.R.-D.)
3 Instituto de Investigación INCLIVA, Hospital Clínico Universitario de Valencia, 46010 Valencia, Spain
4 National Health Research Institute (INIS), Maianga, Luanda P.O. Box 3635, Angola; zoraima.neto@gmail.com (Z.N.); cruzdossantos10@gmail.com (C.S.S.)
5 Centro de Investigação em Saúde de Angola (CISA), Caxito, Luanda P.O. Box 5547, Angola; fortes.elsa@gmail.com (E.F.-G.); miguel.brito@estesl.ipl.pt (M.B.)
6 Instituto Superior Técnico Militar (ISTM), Avenida Deolinda Rodrigues Km 9. Campo Militar do Grafanil, Luanda P.O. Box 5547, Angola
7 Health and Technology Research Center (H & TRC), Escola Superior de Tecnologia da Saúde de Lisboa, Instituto Politécnico de Lisboa, 1990-096 Lisbon, Portugal
8 Centro Nacional de Investigação Científica (CNIC), Avenida Ho Chi Minh, 201, Maianga, Luanda P.O. Box 3635, Angola
9 Global Health and Tropical Medicine (GHTM), Associate Laboratory in Translation and Innovation Towards Global Health, LA-REAL, Instituto de Higiene e Medicina Tropical (IHMT), Universidade NOVA de Lisboa, 1349-008 Lisbon, Portugal
10 Interdisciplinary Center for Research in Animal Health (CIISA), Faculty of Veterinary Medicine, University of Lisbon, 1300-477 Lisbon, Portugal
11 Associate Laboratory for Animal and Veterinary Sciences (AL4AnimalS), 1300-477 Lisbon, Portugal
* Correspondence: ccunha@ihmt.unl.pt (C.C.); claudiaistrate@fmv.ulisboa.pt (C.I.)
† These authors contributed equally to this work.

Abstract: *Rotavirus alphagastroenteritidis* (*R. alphagastroenteritidis*) remains the leading cause of pediatric diarrhea. Although Angola introduced Rotarix®, the human monovalent *R. alphagastroenteritidis* vaccine since 2014 as part of its routine childhood immunization program, no follow-up study has been conducted. The aim of this study was to evaluate the distribution of *R. alphagastroenteritidis* genotypes among children under five years of age, hospitalized with acute gastroenteritis (AGE), after the introduction of the rotavirus vaccine. To achieve this goal, stool samples collected between 2021 and 2022 from children under 5 years of age diagnosed with AGE at six hospitals in Luanda Province were analyzed. The *R. alphagastroenteritidis*-antigen immunochromatographic test (SD Bioline™, Abbott, Chicago, IL, USA) was performed, and 121 positive samples were genotyped. Ten samples were randomly selected for further Sanger sequencing. The results showed that the G9P[6] was the most prevalent genotype (17.3%), followed by G9P[8] (16.5%), G2P[4] (14.9%), G3P[6] (13.2%), G8P[6] (11.5%), and less frequently G12P[8] (9.1%), G1P[6] (4.1%), and G1P[8] (2.5%). The genotype combinations G3P[6], G8P[6], and G12P[8] were detected for the first time in Luanda Province. In conclusion, the emergence of new genotype combinations supports the need for continuous surveillance to identify the trend in *R. alphagastroenteritidis* infection and the emergence of new strains circulating in Luanda Province in the post-vaccination period.

Keywords: *rotavirus alphagastroenteritidis*; genotyping; Rotarix®; Luanda; Angola

1. Introduction

Rotavirus alphagastroenteritidis (*R. alphagastroenteritidis*) is the main causative agent of acute gastroenteritis (AGE) in infants and young children under five years of age and remains the most significant pathogen associated with infant mortality in most low- and middle-income countries (LMICs). It is estimated that 30–50% of childhood diarrheal hospitalizations in LMICs are due to *R. alphagastroenteritidis* infections [1,2]. In 2016, over 128,000 deaths were attributed to *R. alphagastroenteritidis* infections in children under five years of age [3], and about 90% of these fatalities occurred in LMICs, probably due to limited access to health services, lack of hydration therapy, and malnutrition [1]. In 2016, Angola was among the ten LMICs (India, Pakistan, Kenya, Democratic Republic of Congo, Niger, Angola, Ethiopia, Afghanistan, Nigeria, and Chad) with the highest diarrheal burden due to *R. alphagastroenteritidis*, and approximately 100 per 100,000 children died before reaching the age of five [4].

Since 2006, several *R. alphagastroenteritidis* oral live-attenuated vaccines have been licensed and prequalified by WHO for global use. Since then, *R. alphagastroenteritidis* vaccination has been introduced in the childhood immunization programs of more than 120 countries worldwide [5]. In this context, the first two approved *R. alphagastroenteritidis* vaccines were RotaTeq® (RV5; Merck & Co. Inc., Whitehouse Station, NJ, USA) and Rotarix® (RV1; GlaxoSmithKline Biologicals, Rixensart, Belgium). RotaTeq® is a live pentavalent vaccine consisting of a mixture of mono-rearrangements of human and bovine *R. alphagastroenteritidis*, carrying genes encoding for human *R. alphagastroenteritidis* proteins G1, G2, G3, G4, and P[8] inserted into the bovine *R. alphagastroenteritidis* G6P[5] strain, while Rotarix® is a monovalent vaccine derived from a human isolate G1P[8] [6]. The latter was introduced in Angola in 2014. The efficacy/effectiveness of the two vaccines was monitored over the years in both high-income countries and LMICs. Differences between countries have been reported due to various factors, such as malnutrition, breastfeeding, enteric pathogens, histo-blood group antigens, microbiota dysbiosis, and environmental enteropathy [7,8].

Since 2018, two additional vaccines were prequalified by WHO: Rotavac (Bharat Biotech International Ltd., Hyderabad, India) and Rotasiil (Serum Institute of India, Pune, India). Two additional vaccines are used only nationwide in China (Lanzhou lamb *R. alphagastroenteritidis*, manufactured by the Lanzhou Institute of Biomedical Products), and Vietnam (Rotavin-M1, manufactured by Polyvac, Hanoi, Vietnam) (https://www.who.int/teams/immunization-vaccines-and-biologicals/policies/position-papers/rotavirus (accessed on 20 March 2025).

Rotavirus belongs to the *Sedoreoviridae* family and is a large, non-enveloped virus with a triple-layered capsid and a diameter of up to 100 nm. The outer layer contains two capsid proteins, VP4 and VP7, the middle layer consists of the VP6 protein, while the inner core includes the VP2 protein associated with VP1 (RNA-dependent RNA polymerase) and VP3 (viral capping enzyme). The viral genome consists of 11 linear double-stranded RNA (dsRNA) segments, which are packaged entirely in the inner core layer [9]. The genome encodes six structural proteins (VP1-VP4, VP6, and VP7) and six non-structural proteins (NSP1-NSP6). The structural proteins integrated into the virion determine host specificity and mediate entry into the cell. Non-structural proteins, synthesized during infection, are involved in viral replication, pathogenesis, and inhibition of the host innate immune response, and also include the viral enterotoxin (NSP4) [1].

According to the antigenicity of the VP6 intermediate layer, at least ten different rotavirus species have been identified. Among them, *Rotavirus alphagastroenteritidis* (*R. alphagastroenteritidis*), *R. betagastroenteritidis*, *R. tritogastroenteritidis*, and *R. aspergastroenteritidis* infect both humans and other mammalian species [10].

Based on the antigenic and sequence variations of the two outer capsid proteins, VP7 and VP4, the *R. alphagastroenteritidis* strains were categorized into G (glycosylated) and P (protease-sensitive) genotypes, respectively, using a dual classification approach [11]. Although 42 G genotypes and 58 P genotypes have been described in humans and animals, only a few combinations of G and P genotypes are predominantly detected in humans [12]. The most frequently detected human rotavirus genotypes are G1P[8], G2P[4], G3P[8], G4P[8], G8P[8], G9P[8], and G12P[8] [12]. G1P[8] predominates in North America, Europe, and Australia, accounting for more than 70% of *R. alphagastroenteritidis* infections, and is less frequently detected in South America (30%), Asia (30%), and Africa (23%) [13].

The genetic diversity of *R. alphagastroenteritidis* is driven by interspecies transmission and gene rearrangement events, which represent important mechanisms of rotavirus evolution [14]. Humans can be infected by rotaviruses of animal origin, either through direct transmission or through strains resulting from the exchange of one or more genome segments between human and animal rotaviruses [14]. Several evolutionary studies have shown that human rotavirus strains originated from animal strains of independent ancestry. The evolution and diversity of *R. alphagastroenteritidis* strains are thought to be driven by various events that can occur in genome segments, including point mutations and genetic rearrangements through interspecies transmission [15]. The impact of these alterations on the effectiveness of the vaccine has yet to be determined [16].

This study is part of a larger investigation regarding rotavirus infection among children admitted with AGE in several public hospitals in Luanda province, Angola [17], and aims to provide baseline information on *R. alphagastroenteritidis* infection after the introduction of the Rotarix® vaccine in 2014.

2. Materials and Methods

2.1. Study Design

A cross-sectional hospital-based study was conducted from April 2021 to May 2022 at the pediatric emergency and inpatient services of six public hospitals in Luanda Province, namely Luanda General Hospital (H. Luanda), General Hospital Cajueiros of Cazenga (H. Cajueiros of Cazenga), General Hospital of Kilamba Kiaxi (H. Kilamba Kiaxi), Municipal Hospital of Talatona (H. Talatona), Municipal Hospital of Zango (H. Zango), and Municipal Hospital Cacuaco (H. Cacuaco) [17]. This study involved 1251 children under five years of age, hospitalized with AGE. The primary inclusion criteria for participants were defined by diarrhea ($\geq$3 episodes of loose or liquid stools per 24 h) and/or vomiting during a maximum of 7 days.

2.2. Sample Collection and *R. alphagastroenteritidis* Detection

Fecal samples were collected in sterile containers and screened locally for the presence of *R. alphagastroenteritidis* antigens using the WHO-approved SD Bioline™ Rotavirus immunochromatographic rapid test (Abbott, Chicago, IL, USA), following the manufacturer's instructions. Samples were stored on site at 4 °C until they were transported on ice packs to the National Institute for Health Research (INIS) in Luanda, Angola, where genotyping was performed.

2.3. *Genotyping of R. alphagastroenteritidis Strains*

Viral RNA was extracted from stool suspensions at 10% (*w*/*v*) using the NZY Viral RNA Isolation Kit (NZYTech, Lisbon, Portugal) according to the manufacturer's instructions. The RNA was diluted in RNase-free water (60 µL) and stored at −20 °C until further analyses. Synthesis of cDNA was performed by reverse transcription (RT) with random hexamers, using a commercial kit (NZY First-strand cDNA Synthesis Kit, NZYTech, Lisbon, Portugal), according to the manufacturer's instructions. *R. alphagastroenteritidis* G and P genotyping was performed using hemi-nested type specific multiplex PCRs, optimized to detect eight G-types (G1, G2, G3, G4, G8, G9, G10, and G12) and six P-types (P[4], P[6], P[8], P[9], P[10], and P[11]), as described previously [18,19]. The G and P genotypes were assigned according to the amplicon size, as visualized under ultraviolet light after electrophoresis on 2% (*w*/*v*) agarose gels, stained with GreenSafe Premium (NZYTech, Lisbon, Portugal).

2.4. *Sequencing of R. alphagastroenteritidis Strains*

Ten fecal samples were randomly selected for Sanger sequencing of both VP7 and VP4 gene amplicons, with the aim of covering the range of detected G and P genotypes, including non-typable strains. DNA sequencing was performed by STABVIDA Laboratories (Costa da Caparica, Portugal) using the corresponding first-round PCR primers. Complete sequences for both VP4 and VP7 genes were successfully obtained from 4 samples. In 3 samples, only the VP4 gene could be sequenced, while in the remaining 3, only the VP7 gene was recovered. These differences were due to the variability in PCR amplification efficiency and sequence quality among the samples.

2.5. *Phylogenetic Analysis*

The quality of the sequences was manually reviewed and adjusted using BioEdit v7.2.5 software [20]. All sequences were deposited in GenBank (NCBI) under accession numbers PQ139230 to PQ139236 (VP4 gene sequences) and PQ139237 to PQ139243 (VP7 gene sequences).

Phylogenetic trees were constructed using sequences from this study, along with reference sequences retrieved from GenBank. All sequences were aligned using Clustal X 2.1 [21] and matched with GeneDoc 2.7.000 [22]. The software used for phylogenetic tree construction and analysis was MEGA 7.0.23 [23].

The nucleotide substitution model for each tree was selected based on the lowest Bayesian Information Criterion (BIC) score and was also used to calculate the pairwise identity percentages. For the VP4 phylogenetic tree, the Hasegawa Kishino–Yano model was selected, while the Tamura 3-parameter model was used for the VP7 tree. The evolutionary history was inferred using the Maximum Likelihood method [24] with a bootstrap test of 1000 replicates to assess reliability. To further assess genetic variability, nucleotide distance matrices for each genome segment were generated in MEGA 7.0.23 using the p-distance model, a built-in tool of the software.

Additionally, we analyzed differences in the antigenic regions of VP4 and VP7 [25–28] based on the deduced amino acid sequences of the Luanda strains, the Rotarix® and RotaTeq® vaccine strains, and other reference sequences included in the phylogenetic analysis.

2.6. *Statistical Analysis*

Descriptive statistics were used to assess the characteristics of the children enrolled in this study. Data were summarized by number, and absolute (n) and relative (%) frequencies of categorical variables were calculated. To investigate a possible association between age or severity of disease and genotypes (G or P), the children were divided into four age groups (0–6, 7–12, 13–24, >24 months) and 3 AGE groups according to the Vesikari scoring system (mild, moderate, severe), respectively. The association between proportions was assessed with a chi-squared ($\chi 2$) test of independence. A p-value < 0.05 was set as the threshold to assess statistical significance. Data were analyzed using software SPSS version 22 (IBM Corp, Armonk, NY, USA).

2.7. Ethical Considerations

This study was approved by the Independent Ethics Committee of the Faculty of Medicine, Agostinho Neto University, Luanda, Angola (Reference n° 12/2021, 15 January 2021). The parents or legal guardians of each child recruited for the study were informed of the study's objectives and that participation was voluntary. Children were enrolled in the study after obtaining the informed consent form signed by parents or legal guardians.

3. Results

3.1. High Diversity of R. alphagastroenteritidis Strains Detected in Children Hospitalized with AGE in Luanda Province Public Hospitals

Stool samples from 1251 hospitalized children with AGE were screened for *R. alphagastroenteritidis* using an immunochromatographic rapid test. The overall *R. alphagastroenteritidis* detection rate was 57.8% (723/1251) [17]. One hundred and twenty-one *R. alphagastroenteritidis*-positive samples were genotyped, and sequencing confirmation was obtained for ten randomly selected samples, yielding a total of 14 sequences. The most prevalent G genotype was G9 (38.8%), followed by G2 (14.9%), G3 (14.9%), G8 (12.4%), and G12 (9.1%), while the most prevalent P genotypes were P[6] (47.1%), P[8] (28.1%), and P[4] (14.9%) (Table 1).

Table 1. Prevalence of G and P-types in hospitalized children with AGE during the study period (2021–2022).

G-type	N	%
G1	9	7.4
G2	18	14.9
G3	18	14.9
G8	15	12.4
G9	46	38.8
G12	11	9.1
Gnt [a]	3	2.5
Total	121	100
P-type	**N**	**%**
P4	18	14.8
P6	57	47.1
P8	34	28.0
Pnt [b]	12	9.9
Total	121	100

[a] Strains that were non-typable for G; [b] strains that were non-typable for P.

The relative frequency of G and P genotypes during the study period is shown in Figure 1. It can be observed that during the study period (2021–2022), G9P[6] (17.4%) was the most frequently found combination. However, G9P[8] (16.5%), G2P[4] (14.9%), G3P[6] (13.2%), G8P[6] (11.6%), and G12P[8] (9.1%) were also commonly detected. It is worth noting that strains such as G1P[6] (4.1%) and G1P[8] (2.5%), predominantly detected in a previous study from Angola [29] were now less frequently found. Various combinations of G or P non-typable strains were identified with frequencies below 2%.

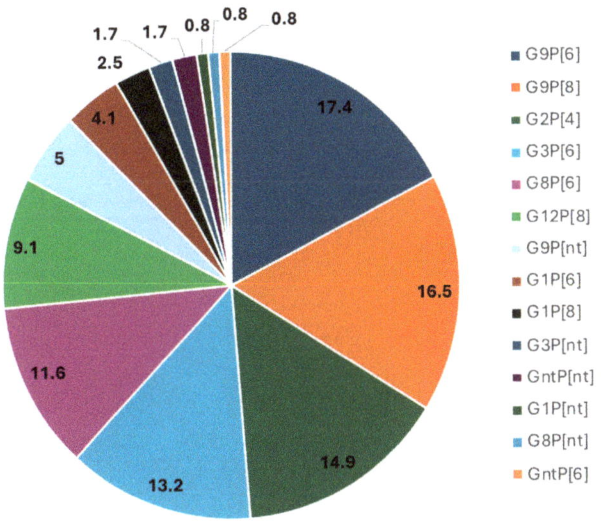

Figure 1. *R. alphagastroenteritidis* strain diversity in hospitals of Luanda Province (2021/2022). *R. alphagastroenteritidis*-positive samples were genotyped using a hemi-nested type-specific multiplex PCR protocol optimized to detect eight G-types (G1, G2, G3, G4, G8, G9, G10, and G11) and six P-types (P[4], P[6], P[8], P[9], P[10]). The results are presented as percentage of each G and P combination in relation to the total number of positive samples (n = 121).

The analysis of frequencies of *R. alphagastroenteritidis* genotypes in each of the six hospitals enrolled in the study showed some tendencies (Table 2). Genotypes G2P[4] and G9P[8] accounted for 68.7% (11/16) of all genotypes detected in H. Cacuaco, G9P[6] was the most frequent genotype in H. Luanda (34.5%; 10/29), G2P[4] and G9P[8] were the most prevalent in H. Zango (51.6%; 16/31), G12P[8] in H. Talatona (41.1%; 7/17), and the G3P[6] and G9P[8] genotypes in H. Kilamba Kiaxi (77.6%; 14/18).

Table 2. Genotypic combinations of *R. alphagastroenteritidis* strains circulating in six hospitals in Luanda Province (2021–2022).

Genotype Combination	Cacuaco n (%)	Luanda n (%)	Zango n (%)	Cajueiros n (%)	Talatona n (%)	K. Kiaxi n (%)	Total n (%)
G1P[6]	0 (0.0)	2 (6.9)	3 (9.7)	0 (0.0)	0 (00.0)	0 (0.0)	5 (4.1)
G1P[8]	0 (0.0)	0 (0.0)	0 (0.0)	0 (0.0)	3 (17.6)	0 (0.0)	3 (2.5)
G1Pnt *	0 (0.0)	1 (3.4)	0 (0.0)	0 (0.0)	0 (0.0)	0 (0.0)	1 (0.8)
G2P[4]	5 (31.2)	3 (10.3)	9 (29.0)	0 (0.0)	1 (5.9)	0 (0.0)	18 (14.9)
G3P[6]	0 (0.0)	2 (6.9)	1 (3.2)	1 (10)	2 (11.8)	10 (55.6)	16 (13.2)
G3Pnt *	0 (0.0)	0 (0.0)	1 (3.2)	0 (0.0)	0 (0.0)	1 (5.6)	2 (1.6)
G8P[6]	1 (6.2)	3 (10.3)	3 (9.7)	4 (40.0)	2 (11.8)	1 (5.6)	14 (11.5)
G8Pnt *	0 (0.0)	1 (3.4)	0 (0.0)	0 (0.0)	0 (0.0)	0 (0.0)	1 (1.7)
G9P[6]	3 (18.8)	10(34.5)	5 (16.1)	1 (10)	1 (5.9)	1 (5.6)	21 (17.3)
G9P[8]	6 (37.5)	3(10.3)	7 (22.6)	0 (0.0)	0 (0.0)	4 (22.0)	20 (16.5)
G9Pnt *	1 (6.3)	0 (0.0)	0 (0.0)	3 (30.0)	1 (5.9)	1 (5.6)	6 (4.9)
G12P[8]	0 (0.0)	2 (6.9)	2 (6.5)	0 (0.0)	7 (41.1)	0 (0.0)	11 (9.1)
* GntP[6]	0 (0.0)	0 (0.0)	0 (0.0)	1 (10)	0 (0.0)	0 (0.0)	1 (0.8)
* GntPnt	0 (0.0)	2 (6.9)	0 (0.0)	0 (0.0)	0 (0.0)	0 (0.0)	2 (1.7)
Total	16 (100)	29 (100)	31 (100)	10 (100)	17 (100)	18 (100)	121 (100)

* Strains that were non-typable for either G-type or P-type.

3.2. Genotype Diversity, Age, and Severity of Disease

We investigated a possible relationship between genotypes and age or severity of disease. A large majority of genotyped samples (95.8%) belonged to children up to 12 months of age, a proportion similar to that found in the whole set of *R. alphagastroenteritidis*-positive cases (98.4%; 712/723) (Table 3). Among G genotypes, G9 was the most frequently detected in children less than 1 year old (35.5%), followed by G2 (14.8%), G3 (14.0%), G8 (12.3%), and G12 (9.0%). In addition, the two most frequent P genotypes in this age group, P[6] and P[8], accounted for 75.2% of all analyzed cases (42.9% P[6] and 32.3% P[8]). A chi-square test of independence showed that there is no significant association between the age group and *R. alphagastroenteritidis* genotypes.

Table 3. Distribution of *R. alphagastroenteritidis* genotypes by age group.

	Age Group (Months)				
Genotype	**0–6 n (%)**	**7–12 n (%)**	**13–24 n (%)**	**>24 n (%)**	**Total**
G1P[6]	3 (3.4)	2 (6.9)	0 (0.0)	0 (0.0)	5 (4.1)
G1P[8]	3 (3.4)	0 (0.0)	0 (0.0)	0 (0.0)	3 (2.5)
G1PN	1 (1.1)	0 (0.0)	0 (0.0)	0 (0.0)	1 (0.8)
G2P[4]	14 (16.1)	4 (13.8)	0 (0.0)	0 (0.0)	18 (14.9)
G3P[6]	12 (13.8)	3 (10.3)	0 (0.0)	1 (33.3)	16 (13.2)
G3PN	2 (2.3)	0 (0.0)	0 (0.0)	0 (0.0)	2 (1.6)
G8P[6]	11 (12.6)	3 (10.3)	0 (0.0)	0 (0.0)	14 (11.5)
G8PN	1 (1.1)	0 (0.0)	0 (0.0)	0 (0.0)	1 (1.7)
G9P[6]	9 (10.3)	8 (27.5)	2 (100)	2 (66.7)	21 (17.3)
G9P[8]	14 (16.1)	6 (20.7)	0 (0.0)	0 (0.0)	20 (16.5)
G9PN	4 (4.6)	2 (6.9)	0 (0.0)	0 (0.0)	6 (4.9)
G12P[8]	10 (11.5)	1 (3.4)	0 (0.0)	0 (0.0)	11 (9.1)
* GntP[6]	1 (1.1)	0 (0.0)	0 (0.0)	0 (0.0)	1 (0.8)
* GntPN	2 (2.9)	0 (0.0)	0 (0.0)	0 (0.0)	2 (1.7)
Total	87 (100)	29 (100)	2 (100)	3 (100)	121 (100)

* Strains that were non-typable for G.

According to the Vesikari scoring system, 90.0% children had severe *R. alphagastroenteritidis* (109/121) (Table 4). In this group, G9 was the predominant G genotype (36.6%), followed by G3 (17.4%), G2 (16.5%), G8 (11.9%), G12 (9.2%), and G1 (7.3%). However, the observed frequency differences were not statistically significant ($p = 0.14$). Moreover, two P genotypes, P[6] (47.1%) and P[8] (28.0%), were found to account for about three quarters of all severe *R. alphagastroenteritidis* cases. The third most frequent P genotype was P[4] (14.9%). A chi-square test of independence was performed, and a statistically significant association was found between the P genotype and severity of disease ($p < 0.001$). However, this association may reflect the predominance of P[6] and P[8] genotypes *in R. alphagastroenteritidis*-infected children, rather than a specific relation to severe diarrhea cases.

Table 4. Distribution of genotype according to the severity of *R. alphagastroenteritidis* AGE using the Vesikari scoring system.

	Severity of Diarrhea			
Genotype	Mild (<7) n (%)	Moderate (7–10) n (%)	Severe (≥11) n (%)	Total n (%)
G1P[6]	0 (0.0)	0 (0.0)	5 (4.5)	5 (4.1)
G1P[8]	0 (0.0)	1 (10.0)	2 (1.8)	3 (2.5)
G1Pnt	0 (0.0)	0 (0.0)	1 (0.9)	1 (0.8)
G2P[4]	0 (0.0)	0 (0.0)	18 (16.5)	18 (14.9)
G3P[6]	0 (0.0)	1 (10.0)	15 (15.6)	16 (13.2)
G3PN	0 (0.0)	0 (0.0)	2 (1.8)	2 (1.6)
G8P[6]	0 (0.0)	2 (20.0)	12 (11.0)	14 (11.5)
G8Pnt	0 (0.0)	0 (0.0)	1 (0.9)	1 (1.7)
G9P[6]	2 (100)	1 (10.0)	18 (16.5)	21 (17.3)
G9P[8]	0 (0.0)	2 (20.0)	18 (16.5)	20 (16.5)
G9PN	0 (0.0)	2 (20.0)	4 (3.6)	6 (4.9)
G12P[8]	0 (0.0)	1 (10.0)	10 (9.2)	11 (9.1)
* GntP[6]	0 (0.0)	0 (0.0)	1 (0.9)	1 (0.8)
* GntPN	0 (0.0)	0 (0.0)	2 (1.8)	2 (1.7)
Total	2 (100)	10 (100)	109 (100)	121 (100)

* Strains that were non-typable for either G-type or P-type.

3.3. Phylogenetic Analysis of *R. alphagastroenteritidis* Strains Identified in Luanda Province Post-Vaccine Introduction

Despite being based on a limited number of sequences, the *R. alphagastroenteritidis* strains analyzed in Luanda Province showed low diversity, clustering within the same lineages of the respective genotypes for both VP4 and VP7.

The phylogenetic analysis of the *R. alphagastroenteritidis* VP4 gene (Figure 2) reveals that the Luanda Province sequences analyzed in this study form monophyletic clusters belonging to lineage III of genotype P[8] and lineage Ia of genotype P[6]. For both genotypes, all sequences included in this study share between 99.8% and 100% identity (Supplementary Figure S1).

Regarding genotype P[8], the results indicate that sequences within lineage III exhibit identity percentages ranging from 79.9% (lineage IV) to 94.7% (lineage II) when compared to reference sequences from other lineages. Notably, lineage III includes sequence CSP10 (KT225724), which was circulating in Angola in 2013. This sequence shares substantial but not complete identity (95.6–95.9%) with the 2021–2022 sequences from the same region (DV66HMZ, DV105HMT, and DV117HMT) [29]. Additionally, these sequences display 92.1–92.3% and 86.4–86.7% identity with the vaccine strains RotaTeq® and Rotarix® (the vaccine administered in Angola), respectively.

For genotype P[6], the phylogenetic analysis shows that sequences DV68HKK, DV114HKK, DV120HKK, and DV177HKK cluster with a strain that was circulating in the region in 2012 (C27, KT225683), sharing 97.5% identity [29]. In contrast, identity analysis of the 2021 Luanda Province sequences with other lineages indicates a significant genetic divergence from subgroup Ib/c (86.6%) and even greater divergence from reference sequences of other lineages, with identity percentages ranging from 54.3% (lineage II) to 73.9% (lineage IV) (Supplementary Figure S2).

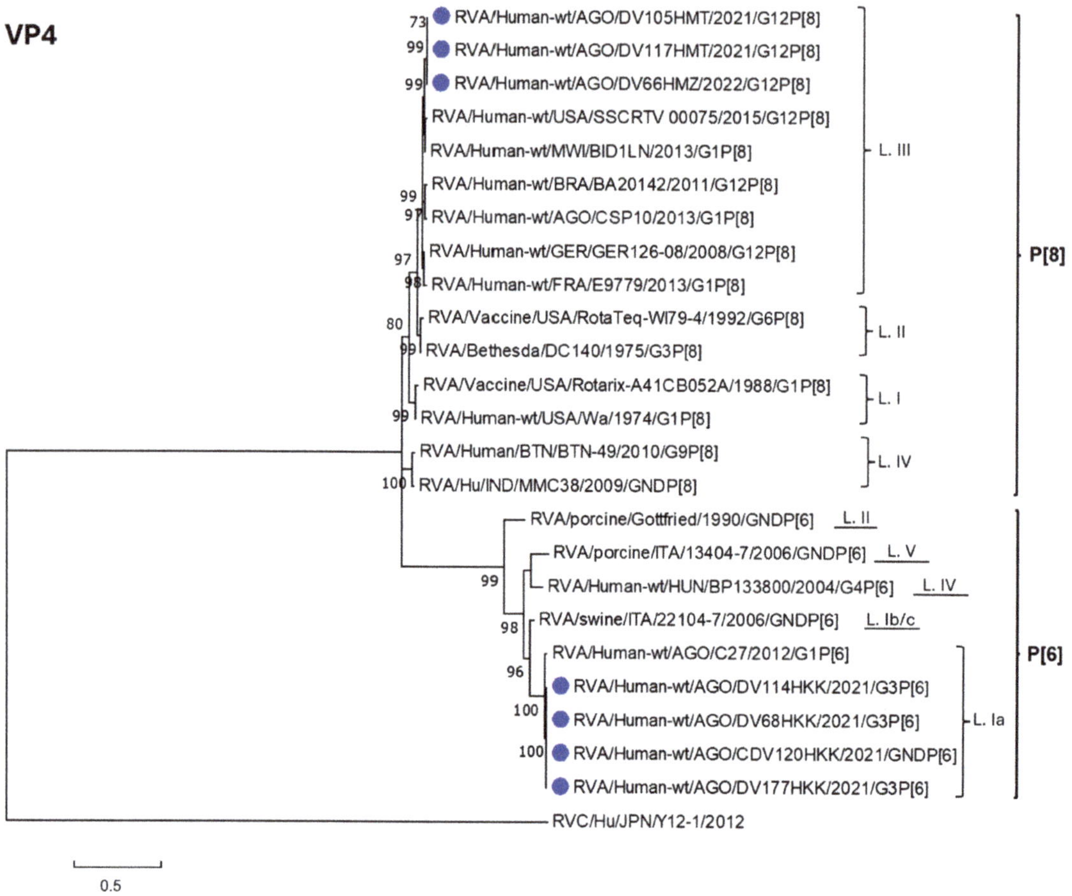

Figure 2. Molecular phylogenetic analysis by Maximum Likelihood (ML) method. The ML tree with the highest log likelihood (−3898.30) is shown. The percentage of trees in which the associated taxa clustered together is shown next to the branches. Initial tree(s) for the heuristic search were obtained automatically by applying neighbor joining and BioNJ algorithms to a matrix of pairwise distances estimated using the Maximum Composite Likelihood (MCL) approach, and then selecting the topology with superior log likelihood value. A discrete Gamma distribution was used to model evolutionary rate differences among sites (5 categories (+G, parameter = 2.0878)). The rate variation model allowed for some sites to be evolutionarily invariable ([+I], 12.52% sites). The tree is drawn to scale, with branch lengths measured in the number of substitutions per site. The analysis involved 25 nucleotide sequences. All positions containing gaps and missing data were removed. There was a total of 563 positions in the final dataset. Evolutionary analyses were conducted in MEGA7 [24]. RVA = *R. alphagastroenteritidis*. Blue dots indicate *R. alphagastroenteritidis* sequences obtained from patients' samples and analyzed in this study.

The VP7 gene dendrogram (Figure 3) illustrates the clustering of Luanda Province sequences into different genotypes (G3, G8, G9, and G12). The 2021–2022 Luanda Province sequences belonging to genotype G3 (DV68HKK, DV177HKK, and DV114HKK) share 99.1–99.7% identity and cluster within lineage I alongside the RotaTeq® vaccine strain, although with a high but incomplete identity (90.9–92.2%). The 2022 Luanda Province G8 sequences (DV34HECJ and DV540HGL) are identical to each other and exhibit high similarity (98.2%) with sequence CSMI10 (KT225669), belonging to a strain that circulated in Angola in 2012 [29]. Regarding sequence DV117HMT, classified as genotype G12, it clusters within lineage II and shares 95.6% identity with sequence AH6 (KT225672) from lineage III, which corresponds to a strain that was also circulating in Angola in 2012 [29]. Lastly, the 2022 sequence DV72HMCC clusters within lineage VI of genotype G9, distinct from sequence C84 (KT225671), which belongs to a strain found in Angola in 2012 that clusters within lineage III [29].

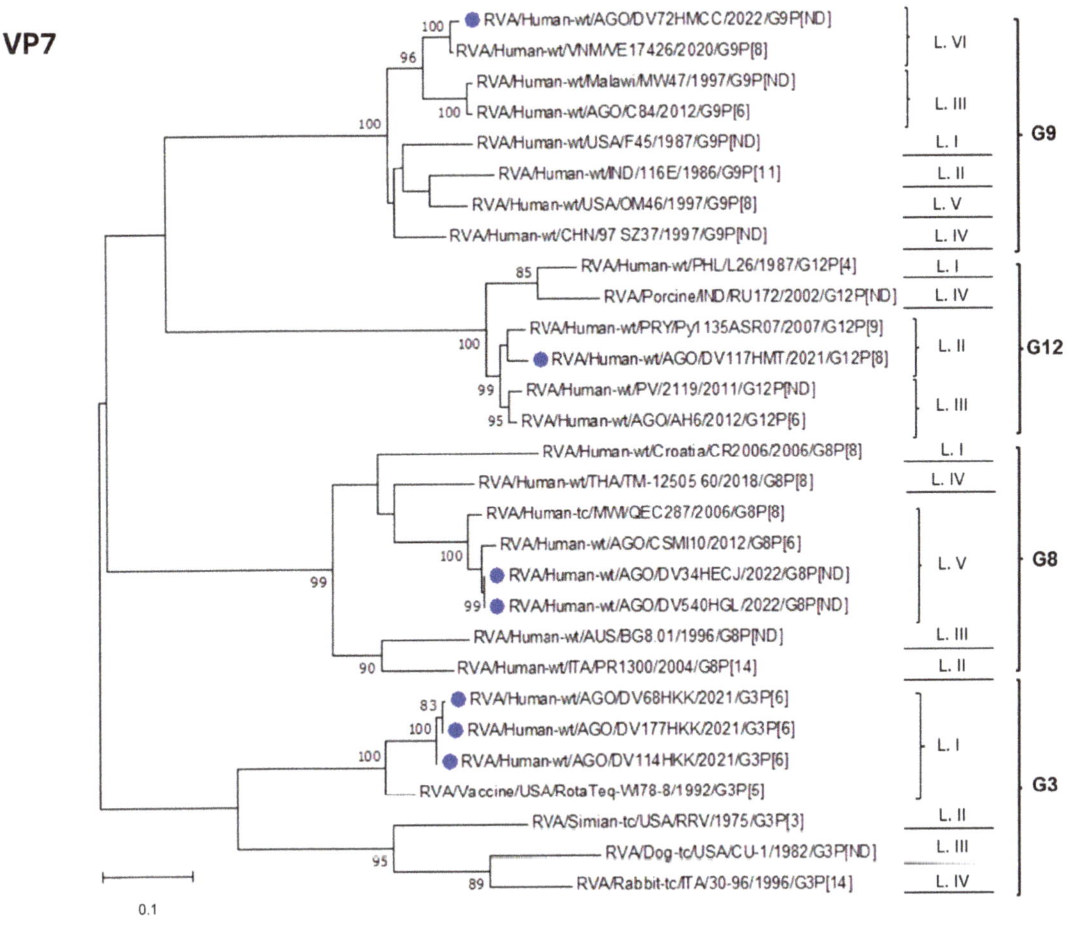

Figure 3. Molecular Phylogenetic analysis by Maximum Likelihood (ML) method. The ML tree with the highest log likelihood (−2981.70) is shown. The percentage of trees in which the associated taxa clustered together is shown next to the branches. Initial tree(s) for the heuristic search were obtained automatically by applying neighbor joining and BioNJ algorithms to a matrix of pairwise distances estimated using the Maximum Composite Likelihood (MCL) approach, and then selecting the topology with superior log likelihood value. A discrete Gamma distribution was used to model evolutionary rate differences among sites (five categories (+G, parameter = 1.5436)). The rate variation model allowed for some sites to be evolutionarily invariable ([+I], 26.98% sites). The tree is drawn to scale, with branch lengths measured as the number of substitutions per site. The analysis involved 29 nucleotide sequences. All positions containing gaps and missing data were eliminated. There was a total of 354 positions in the final dataset. Evolutionary analyses were conducted in MEGA7 [23]. RVA = *R. alphagastroenteritidis*. Blue dots indicate *R. alphagastroenteritidis* sequences obtained from patients' samples and analyzed in this study.

3.4. Comparison of the Deduced Antigenic Region of VP4 (VP8 *) and VP7

Tables 5 and 6 show the positions of the deduced amino acid sequences corresponding to the antigenic regions of VP4 (VP8 *: 8-1, 8-2, 8-3, and 8-4) and VP7 (7-1a, 7-1b, and 7-2), respectively. These tables provide a detailed overview of the amino acid composition of these regions for each analyzed sample.

Concerning the VP4 (VP8 *) epitope, we identified seven amino acids conserved across all strains (Table 5): D100, S188, T190, and L103 in region 8-1; T180 and A183 in region 8-2; and N132 in region 8-3. This homology represents 28% of the epitope (7/25 aa).

Within the same genotype, all Luanda Province sequences exhibited 100% similarity in the antigenic region. Furthermore, our results show that P[8] genotype sequences display greater epitope conservation compared to those of the P[6] genotype sequences (60% and 44%, respectively). Finally, sequences belonging to the same lineage displayed higher homology when compared to sequences assigned to other lineages.

Regarding the P[8] genotype, Luanda Province sequences differed by three amino acids compared to other reference sequences of the same lineage (lineage III), namely in positions 194, 113, and 89. Specifically, we observed a N194D substitution in comparison with strains GER126-08 (Germany, 2008, genotype G12P[8]) and E9779 (France, 2013, genotype G1P[8]); a N113D substitution was observed in comparison with strains CSP10 (Angola, 2013, genotype G1P[8]) and BA20142 (Brazil, 2011, genotype G12P[8]); and a T89N substitution was found in comparison with all other P[8] strains, including the Rotarix® vaccine strain (lineage I of genotype P[8]).

Overall, Luanda P[8] strains exhibited 24% variability in the antigenic region compared to the Rotarix® vaccine strain. Specifically, we identified the following amino acid substitutions: D150E (both acidic), G195N (both polar uncharged), N125S (both polar uncharged), R131S (acidic and polar uncharged, respectively), D135N (acidic and polar uncharged, respectively), and T89N (both polar uncharged).

For the P[6] genotype, Luanda Province strains differed by a single amino acid P114N (nonpolar and polar, respectively) compared to strain C27 (G1P[6] genotype), which was circulating in Angola in 2012. In comparison with the Rotarix® vaccine strain, Luanda Province P[6] strains exhibited 60% variability in the antigenic region.

Concerning the VP7 epitope, we performed a comparison of the antigenic region among the deduced amino acid sequences of the protein, as shown in Table 6. The limited nucleotide sequence lengths obtained for VP7 in samples DV540HGL (411 nt) and DV34HECJ (409 nt) did not allow for analysis of the corresponding complete antigenic regions. Additionally, sequences for the G1P[8] genotype in Luanda Province could not be obtained for comparison with the Rotarix® vaccine strain.

Overall, the results show 20.7% homology in the VP7 epitope across all sequences analyzed, including amino acids T91, W98, Q104, and K291 from region 7-1a; Q201 from region 7-1b; and S190 and G264 from region 7-2.

Sequences from the same genotype exhibit slightly higher, though not complete, homology (82.8% for the G12 and G9 genotypes and 79.3% for the G8 genotype). The lowest homology was observed among G3 genotype sequences (62.1%).

Considering the number of missing positions due to nucleotide sequence length limitations, the variability in the VP7 epitope between the Luanda Province sequences and the Rotarix® vaccine strain was 60.7% (G12 strains), 48.3% (G3 strains), 45.5% (G8 strains), and 53.6% (G9 strains).

Table 5. VP4 (VP8 *) antigenic regions (8-1, 8-2, 8-3, and 8-4), showing the amino acids present in each strain included in the study.

Lineage		Strain	VP4 (VP8 *) EPITOPE																							
			8-1											8-2		8-3									8-4		
			100	146	148	150	188	190	192	193	194	195	196	180	183	113	114	115	116	125	131	132	133	135	87	88	89
P[8]	III	**RVA/Hu/AGO/DV105HMT/2021/G12P[8]**	D	S	Q	D	S	T	N	L	N	G	I	T	A	N	P	V	D	N	R	N	D	D	N	T	T
		RVA/Hu/AGO/DV117HMT/2021/G12P[8]	.	.	.	.	.	.	.	.	.	.	.	.	.	.	.	.	.	.	.	.	.	.	.	.	.
		RVA/Hu/AGO/DV66HMZ/2022/G12P[8]	.	.	.	.	.	.	.	.	.	.	.	.	.	.	.	.	.	.	.	.	.	.	.	.	.
		RVA/Hu/MWI/BID1LN/2013/G1P[8]	.	.	.	.	.	.	.	.	.	.	.	.	.	.	.	.	.	.	.	.	.	.	.	.	N
		RVA/Hu/USA/SSCRTV 00075/2015/G12P[8]	.	.	.	.	.	.	.	.	.	.	.	.	.	.	.	.	.	.	.	.	.	.	.	.	N
		Hu/GER126-08/GER/2008/G12P[8]	.	.	.	.	.	.	.	.	D	.	.	.	.	.	.	.	.	.	.	.	.	.	.	.	N
		RVA/Hu/AGO/CSP10/2013/G1P[8]	.	.	.	.	.	.	.	.	.	.	.	.	.	D	.	.	.	.	.	.	.	.	.	.	N
		RVA/Hu/BRA/BA20142/2011/G12P[8]	.	.	.	.	.	.	.	.	.	.	.	.	.	D	.	.	.	.	.	.	.	.	.	.	N
		RVA/Hu/FRA/E9779/2013/G1P[8]	.	.	.	.	.	.	.	.	D	.	.	.	.	.	.	.	.	.	.	.	.	.	.	.	N
	IV	RVA/Hu/BTN-49/BTN/2010/G9P[8]	.	.	.	E	.	.	D	.	T	S	.	.	.	D	.	.	.	S	.	.	.	N	.	.	N
		RVA/Hu/IND/MMC38/2009/GNDP[8]	.	G	.	E	.	.	D	.	T	S	.	.	.	D	.	.	.	S	.	.	.	N	.	.	N
	II	Vac/RotaTeq-WI79-4/USA/1992/G6P[8]	.	.	.	E	.	.	.	.	.	D	.	.	.	.	.	.	.	.	.	.	.	.	.	.	N
		RVA/Bethesda/DC140/1975/G3P[8]	.	.	.	E	.	.	.	.	.	D	.	.	.	.	.	.	.	.	.	.	.	.	.	.	N
	I	Vac/Rotarix/USA/2009/G1P[8]	.	.	.	E	.	.	.	.	.	N	.	.	.	.	.	.	.	S	S	.	.	N	.	.	N
		RVA/Hu/USA/Wa/1974/G1P[8]	.	.	.	E	.	.	.	.	.	N	.	.	.	.	.	.	.	S	S	.	.	N	.	.	N
P[6]	II	RVA/porcine/Gottfried/1990/GNDP[6]	.	N	N	D	.	.	.	.	P	D	V	.	.	P	S	Q	.	V	E	.	S	.	I	N	K
	Ia	**RVA/Hu/AGO/DV114HKK/2021/G3P[6]**	.	.	S	E	.	.	.	.	S	E	V	.	.	T	S	Q	S	T	E	.	N	S	T	N	Q
		RVA/Hu/AGO/DV68HKK/2021/G3P[6]	.	.	S	E	.	.	.	.	S	E	V	.	.	T	S	Q	S	T	E	.	N	S	T	N	Q
		RVA/Hu/AGO/DV177HKK/2021/G3P[6]	.	.	S	E	.	.	.	.	S	E	V	.	.	T	S	Q	S	T	E	.	N	S	T	N	Q
		RVA/Hu/AGO/CDV120HKK/2021/GND P[6]	.	.	S	E	.	.	.	.	S	E	V	.	.	T	S	Q	S	T	E	.	N	S	T	N	Q
		RVA/Hu/AGO/C27/2012/G1P[6]	.	.	S	E	.	.	.	.	S	E	V	.	.	T	N	Q	S	T	E	.	N	S	T	N	Q
	Ib/c	RVA/swine/ITA/22104-7/2006/GNDP[6]	.	.	S	E	.	.	.	.	S	E	V	.	.	T	S	Q	S	T	E	.	N	N	T	N	Q
	IV	RVA/Hu/HUN/BP133800/2004/G4P[6]	.	N	S	E	.	.	.	.	S	E	.	.	.	T	N	Q	S	T	E	.	S	N	T	N	Q
	V	RVA/porcine/ITA/13404-7/2006/GNDP[6]	.	N	S	E	.	.	.	.	P	D	.	.	.	T	N	Q	S	M	E	.	N	S	T	N	Q

RVA = *R. alphagastroenteritidis*.

Table 6. VP7 antigenic regions (7-1a, 7-1b, and 7-2), showing the amino acids present in each strain included in the study.

Lineage		Strain	VP7 EPITOPE																												
			7-1a														7-1b						7-2								
			87	91	94	96	97	98	99	100	104	123	125	129	130	291	201	211	212	213	238	242	143	145	146	147	148	190	217	221	264
G12	II	**RVA/Hu/AGO/DV117HMT/2021/G12P[8]**	S	T	T	P	D	W	T	N	Q	D	S	V	D	...	Q	D	V	T	N	N	Q	Q	N	S	L	S	E	A	G
		RVA/Hu/Py1135ASR07/PRY/2007/G12P[9]	.	.	.	.	.	.	.	.	.	.	A	.	.	K	.	.	.	.	.	.	.	.	.	.	.	.	.	.	.
	III	RVA/Hu/2119/PV/2011/G12P[ND]	.	.	.	.	.	.	.	.	.	.	.	.	.	...	.	.	.	.	.	.	.	.	.	.	.	.	.	.	.
		RVA/Hu/AGO/AH6/2012/G12P[6]	.	.	.	.	.	.	.	.	.	.	.	.	.	...	.	.	.	.	.	.	.	.	.	.	.	.	.	.	.
	I	Hu/L26/PHL/1987/G12P[4]	N	.	.	.	.	.	.	H	.	.	A	.	N	K	.	.	.	A	.	.	.	.	.	.	.	.	.	.	.
	IV	Po/RU172/IND/2002/G12PX	N	.	.	.	.	.	.	.	.	.	A	.	.	K	.	.	.	A	.	.	.	.	.	.	.	.	.	.	.
G1		**Vac/Rotarix/USA/2009/G1P[8]**	T	.	N	G	E	.	K	D	.	S	V	.	.	K	.	N	.	D	.	T	K	D	Q	N	.	.	M	N	.
G3	I	Vac/RotaTeq-W178-8/USA/1992/G3P[5]	T	.	N	N	S	.	K	D	.	.	A	.	.	K	.	.	A	N	K	D	K	D	A	T	.	.	.	.	.
		RVA/Hu/AGO/DV114HKK/2021/G3P[6]	T	.	N	N	S	.	K	.	.	.	A	.	.	K	.	.	T	N	.	.	K	D	V	T	.	.	.	D	.
		RVA/Hu/AGO/DV177HKK/2021/G3P[6]	T	.	N	N	S	.	K	.	.	.	A	.	.	K	.	.	T	N	.	.	K	D	V	T	.	.	.	D	.
		RVA/Hu/AGO/DV68HKK/2021/G3P[6]	T	.	N	N	S	.	K	.	.	.	A	.	.	...	.	.	T	N	.	.	K	D	V	T	.	.	.	D	.
	II	RVA/Simian/USA/RRV/1975/G3P[3]	T	.	N	N	S	.	K	D	.	.	A	.	.	K	.	.	T	A	D	A	K	D	A	T	.	.	.	.	.
	III	RVA/Dog/USA/CU-1/1982/G3P[ND]	T	.	N	N	S	.	K	D	.	.	A	.	.	K	.	.	.	S	D	T	K	D	A	A	.	.	.	T	.
	IV	RVA/Rabbit/ITA/30-96/1996/G3P[14]	T	.	N	N	S	.	K	D	.	.	V	.	.	K	.	N	A	A	D	A	K	D	A	A	.	.	.	.	.
G8	V	**RVA/Hu/AGO/DV540HGL/2022/G8P[ND]**	...	...	...	...	...	...	...	...	...	...	...	...	...	K	.	.	T	.	.	T	...	...	...	...	...	.	.	.	.
		RVA/Hu/AGO/DV34HECJ/2022/G8P[ND]	...	...	...	...	...	...	...	...	...	...	...	...	...	K	.	.	T	.	.	T	...	...	...	...	...	.	.	.	.
		RVA/Hu/AGO/CSMI10/2012/G8P[6]	A	.	A	N	S	.	K	D	.	.	A	I	N	...	.	.	T	.	.	T	K	N	T	N	S	.	.	.	.
		RVA/Hu/MWI/QEC287/2006/G8P[8]	A	.	A	S	S	.	K	D	.	.	A	I	N	...	.	.	T	.	.	T	K	N	A	N	S	.	.	.	.
	I	RVA/Hu/Croatia/CR2006/2006/G8P[8]	T	.	A	S	S	.	K	E	.	.	A	I	N	K	.	.	T	.	.	T	K	S	A	N	S	.	.	.	.
	II	RVA/Hu/ITA/PR1300/2004/G8P[14]	V	.	A	S	S	.	K	D	.	.	A	I	N	K	.	.	T	.	.	T	K	N	A	N	S	.	.	.	.
	III	RVA/Hu/AUS/BG8.01/1996/G8P[ND]	V	.	A	S	S	.	K	D	.	.	A	I	N	K	.	.	T	.	.	T	K	N	A	N	S	.	.	.	.
	IV	RVA/Hu/THA/TM-12505_60/2018/G8P[8]	T	.	A	S	S	.	K	D	.	.	A	I	N	...	.	.	T	.	.	T	K	N	A	D	S	.	.	.	.

Table 6. *Cont.*

G9	VI	**RVA/Hu/AGO/DV72HMCC/2022/G9P[ND]**	T	.	G	T	E	.	K	.	.	.	A	I	.	...	.	N	T	A	D	.	K	D	S	T	.	.	.	S	.
		RVA/Hu/VNM/VE17426/2020/G9P[8]	T	.	G	T	E	.	K	.	.	.	A	I	.	K	.	N	T	A	D	.	K	D	S	T	.	.	.	S	.
	I	RVA/Hu/USA/F45/1987/G9P[ND]	A	.	G	T	E	.	K	D	.	.	A	I	.	K	.	N	T	A	D	T	K	D	S	T	.	.	.	S	.
	II	RVA/Hu/IND/116E/1986/G9P[11]	I	.	G	T	E	.	K	G	.	.	A	I	.	K	.	N	T	A	D	.	K	N	S	T	.	.	.	N	.
	III	RVA/Hu/Malawi/MW47/1997/G9P[ND]	T	.	G	T	E	.	K	D	.	.	A	I	.	K	.	N	T	A	D	.	K	D	S	T	.	.	.	S	.
		RVA/Hu/AGO/C84/2012/G9P[6]	T	.	G	T	E	.	K	D	.	.	A	I	.	...	.	N	T	A	D	.	K	D	S	T	.	.	.	S	.
	IV	RVA/Hu/CHN/97'SZ37/1997/G9P[ND]	T	.	G	T	E	.	K	D	.	.	A	I	.	K	.	N	T	A	D	.	K	D	S	T	.	.	.	S	.
	V	RVA/Hu/USA/OM46/1997/G9P[8]	T	.	G	T	E	.	K	D	.	.	A	I	.	K	.	N	T	A	D	.	K	D	S	T	.	.	.	S	.

RVA = *R. alphagastroenteritidis.*

On the other hand, the sample DV117HMT (G12P[8] genotype), found in Luanda Province in 2021–2022, showed no changes in the antigenic region compared to strain AH6, which circulated in Angola in 2012. Again, considering the absence of amino acid data from the Luanda Province G8 genotype strains (DV540HGL and DV34HECJ), which were found in 2021–2022, a comparison with strain CSMI10 (Angola 2012, G8P[6] genotype), belonging to the same lineage (lineage V), showed 100% homology (comparison of 10 positions in the antigenic region). Finally, the sample DV72HMCC (lineage VI of the G9P[ND] genotype), found in Luanda Province in 2021–2022, presented a single amino acid change, N100D (polar uncharged to acidic) compared to sample C84 (Angola 2012, the G9P[6] genotype).

4. Discussion

This study provides a significant update on the molecular epidemiology of *R. alphagastroenteritidis* circulating strains among children under five years of age, admitted with AGE at pediatric emergency services after the introduction of Rotarix® vaccine in 2014. Our results showed a wide diversity of genotype combinations, a major shift in the distribution of genotypes during the study period, and a different dynamic of strains after the introduction of Rotarix® into the Angolan Expanded Program for Immunization.

Some of the identified *R. alphagastroenteritidis* genotype combinations, G1P[8], G2P[4], G9P[8], and G12P[8], have been previously reported as among the six most common strains detected in humans globally (i.e., G1P[8], G2P[4], G3P[8], G4P[8], G9P[8], and G12P[8]) [30]. However, some uncommon genotypes thought to gain a growing epidemiological relevance in Africa [31], such as G8P[6], were detected with non-negligible frequencies (11.6%). Moreover, some genotypes detected here, such as G3P[6] (13.2%) and G9P[6] (17.6%), have been less commonly reported in Africa to date [31,32].

In our previous studies regarding the molecular epidemiology of *R. alphagastroenteritidis* in four provinces of Angola in 2011–2012 [29] and in the Northwestern Bengo Province in 2012–2013 [33], genotype G1P[8], which is also part of the vaccine makeup currently administered in Angola, was the most often detected, with frequencies of 50% and 47.2%, respectively. Nonetheless, in the present study, the frequency of detection of this genotype was strikingly low (2.5%). It is likely that the introduction of the vaccine or natural temporal fluctuations created selective pressure, driving the observed change in the circulating genotypes, a phenomenon reported in other geographic regions. This drastic reduction in the circulation of the G1P[8] strain with concomitant replacement by novel emerging *R. alphagastroenteritidis* strains, such as G3P[8], was earlier reported in Italy, in 2018–2019, after the introduction of the Rotarix® vaccine [34]. In the two above-mentioned studies from Angola [29,33], genotype G1P[6] was the second most prevalent, with frequencies around 29%. Herein, the detection rate of this genotype dramatically decreased to 4.1%. An opposite tendency was observed with genotype G9P[6], which was among the less commonly detected genotypes in 2012 (1.7%) [29] and has become the most prevalent genotype in Luanda Province after the introduction of the Rotarix® vaccine, with a frequency of 17.3%. Notably, the genotype G3P[6], not identified in previous studies in Angola, was now among the most commonly detected genotypes (13.2%). It is important to note that, similarly to our data, earlier studies from Mozambique [35] and Malawi [36] also reported an emergence of G3 strains after the introduction of the Rotarix® vaccine.

We detected six G-types of *R. alphagastroenteritidis* (G1, G2, G3, G8, G9, and G12), with G9 being the most frequent genotype in all hospitals (38.8%). Overall, a shift was observed from globally common G-types (G1–G4, G9, G12) to G9, G3, G8, and G12. The decline in the G1-type (predominant in the pre-vaccination era) and the dominance of G9 was also acknowledged in other African countries, such as South Africa [30]. As for the P-type, P[6] was recorded in high proportion at all study sites, followed by P[8] and P[4]. Genotype P[6] was now found as the most frequent (47.1%), although P[8] and P[4] were also observed with a significant frequency (28% and 14.9%, respectively). The three P genotypes, P[4], P[6], and P[8] accounted for about 90% of all circulating *R. alphagastroenteritidis* strains detected after introduction of the Rotarix® vaccine.

When comparing the most prevalent G/P combinations before and after the introduction of Rotarix®, G9P[6] was the most prevalent genotype combination in this post-vaccination study period, while G1P[8] was the most prevalent genotype combination in the pre-vaccination period [29,33]. The genotype combination G9P[6] can be detected worldwide, namely in countries and regions where the vaccine has been introduced [31,37]. However, a different tendency was reported in early epidemiological studies performed in India [38]. These studies showed high detection rates of G9P[6], leading to the inclusion of this genotype in the development of the first Indian rotavirus vaccine.

The reduced detection rate of the G1P[8] genotype combination may be attributed to the introduction of the vaccine, since Rotarix® is a monovalent vaccine specific to this genotype. Similarly to Angola, other countries that have implemented vaccination programs with the Rotarix® vaccine also reported a decline in the circulation of G1P[8] genotype combinations. This post-vaccination tendency can be illustrated by the reduction in G1P[8] frequencies and the simultaneous increase in the detection rate of other non-G1P[8] combinations in South Africa [39], as well as the rise in heterotypic strains, such as G2P[4] in Brasil [40].

In the VP4 (VP8 *) epitope, seven out of 25 amino acids (D100, L103, N132, T180, A183, S188, and T190) were found to be conserved in all strains (28% homology). Both P[6] and P[8] genotypes displayed high homology with a strain circulating in Angola in 2012, as well as with other reference genotypes. They differed only by 1 and 3 amino acids, respectively, in the VP4 (VP8 *) epitope. In addition, further comparison of the P[6] and P[8] epitopes of the Luanda Province strains with the Rotarix® vaccine strain showed 60% and 24%, respectively, variability in the antigenic region.

With regard to the VP7 epitope, we could not obtain sequences for the G1P[8] genotype, and for two samples, DV540HGL and DV34HECJ, the length of the obtained sequence was limited (409 nt and 411 nt, respectively). Overall, the analysis of the deduced amino acid sequences showed 20.7% homology in the VP7 epitope. Furthermore, when compared to the Rotarix® vaccine strain, the variability in the VP7 epitope displayed by Luanda Province sequences was 48.3% (G3 strains), 45.5% (G8 strains), 53.6% (G9 strains), and 60.7% (G12 strains).

Given the limited number of sequences analyzed, any interpretation of amino acid changes remains speculative. Nonetheless, substitutions involving residues with differing chemical properties—such as nonpolar, polar, and charged amino acids—in key regions of VP4 (VP8) and VP7 were observed, which may suggest potential conformational alterations in antigenic epitopes. However, the biological relevance of these putative changes is uncertain and requires confirmation through analysis of a larger dataset.

The detected changes in amino acids in the epitope regions of circulating strains, when compared to those of the vaccine strain, may also be indicative of the presence of a selective immune pressure. Although speculative, this pressure could accelerate the emergence of new *R. alphagastroenteritidis* strains capable of evading the immune response. Monitoring this emergence in the post-vaccination era is a task of utmost relevance to reduce the burden of *R. alphagastroenteritidis* infection, especially in LMIC.

This study has some limitations that should be considered. First, because it was a cross-sectional study, it was not possible to establish causal relationships between the detected genotypes and clinical severity. Second, our sampling was carried out only in public hospitals in the province of Luanda, which may not reflect the situation in other regions of Angola. Third, genetic analysis was performed on a limited number of samples, which may not capture the full diversity of circulating strains. Finally, the use of rapid tests for the initial detection of *R. alphagastroenteritidis* may have reduced sensitivity, especially in cases with low viral load. Nevertheless, our findings are essential for evaluating the effectiveness of childhood immunization against rotavirus, as well as guiding public policies for vaccination and control of gastroenteritis in Angola.

5. Conclusions

This is the first report to describe the circulation of *R. alphagastroenteritidis* genotypes in Luanda Province, Angola, and revealed a change in the circulating genotypes after the introduction of the Rotarix® vaccine in 2014. However, due to the short surveillance period, it is unclear whether the changes observed are due to the introduction of the vaccine or are a consequence of the natural variation of the strain. In addition, the emergence of unusual strains such as G9P[8], G3P[6], and G12P[8] has also been observed, which supports the need for continued genomic and epidemiological surveillance in Luanda to monitor changes due to possible vaccine pressure and, consequently, asses their effect on vaccine efficacy.

Supplementary Materials: The following supporting information can be downloaded at https://www.mdpi.com/article/10.3390/v17060858/s1, Figure S1: Nucleotide distance matrix for VP4 gene. The number of base substitutions per site between sequences are shown. Standard error estimate(s) are shown above the diagonal and were obtained by a bootstrap procedure (1000 replicates). The analysis involved 25 nucleotide sequences. There was a total of 563 positions. Evolutionary analyses were conducted in MEGA7. Figure S2: Nucleotide distance matrix for VP7 gene. The number of base substitutions per site from between sequences are shown. Standard error estimate(s) are shown above the diagonal and were obtained by a bootstrap procedure (1000 replicates). The analysis involved 29 nucleotide sequences. There was a total of 354 positions. Evolutionary analyses were conducted in MEGA7.

Author Contributions: Conceptualization: C.I., Z.N. and C.C. Laboratory procedures were performed by D.G.V., E.F.-G., C.S.S. and M.B. Methodology: C.I., M.L. and Z.N. The data were analyzed by D.G.V., M.L., C.S.-B., J.R.-D., C.C. and C.I. Validation: E.F.-G., M.B., C.I., C.C., Z.N. and M.L. Formal analysis: C.I., M.L., C.C. and C.S.-B. Investigation: C.I. and D.G.V. Resources: D.G.V., Z.N., E.F.-G. and M.B. Data curation: M.L. and D.G.V. Writing—original draft: D.G.V., C.S.-B., M.L., M.B., E.F.-G., Z.N., C.S.S., J.R.-D., C.C. and C.I. Writing—review and editing: J.R.-D., C.S.-B., C.S.S., C.C. and C.I. Visualization: C.I. and C.C. Supervision: C.I., C.C. and Z.N. Project administration: Z.N. and E.F.-G. Funding acquisition: D.G.V. and E.F.-G. All authors have read and agreed to the published version of the manuscript.

Funding: This research was funded by Abbott Rapid Diagnostics Group, the National Health Research Institute (INIS), Luanda, Angola, the Centro de Investigação em Saúde de Angola (CISA), Angola, and the Gulbenkian Foundation, Lisbon, Portugal. The study sponsors had no role in the design of this study.

Institutional Review Board Statement: This study was conducted according to the ethical principles of biomedical research involving human subjects established in the Declaration of Helsinki (1975). Approval was obtained from the Ethics Committee of Faculty of Medicine, Agostinho Neto University (UAN), Luanda, Angola (Deliberation nº 12/2021, 15 January 2021).

Informed Consent Statement: Informed consent was obtained from all subjects involved in the study.

Data Availability Statement: All the sequences obtained in the present work are available in the GenBank repository under accession numbers PQ139230 to PQ139236 (VP4 gene sequences) and PQ139237 to PQ139243 (VP7 gene sequences). Any remaining data are available on request from the authors.

Acknowledgments: The authors thank the Abbott Group for the support that made it possible to carry out the presented work. We also thank all employees of the six hospitals in Luanda Province, and especially the clinical staff, for their support and collaboration.

Conflicts of Interest: The authors declare no conflicts of interest.

References

1. Crawford, S.E.; Ramani, S.; Tate, J.E.; Parashar, U.D.; Svensson, L.; Hagbom, M.; Franco, M.A.; Greenberg, H.B.; O'Ryan, M.; Kang, G.; et al. Rotavirus infection. *Nat. Rev. Dis. Primers* **2017**, *3*, 17083. [CrossRef] [PubMed]
2. Jampanil, N.; Kumthip, K.; Maneekarn, N.; Khamrin, P. Genetic Diversity of Rotaviruses Circulating in Pediatric Patients and Domestic Animals in Thailand. *Trop. Med. Infect. Dis.* **2023**, *8*, 347. [CrossRef]
3. Troeger, C.; Khalil, I.A.; Rao, P.C.; Cao, S.; Blacker, B.F.; Ahmed, T.; Armah, G.; Bines, J.E.; Brewer, T.G.; Colombara, D.V.; et al. Rotavirus Vaccination and the Global Burden of Rotavirus Diarrhea Among Children Younger Than 5 Years. *JAMA Pediatr.* **2018**, *172*, 958–965. [CrossRef]
4. Tate, J.E.; Burton, A.H.; Boschi-Pinto, C.; Parashar, U.D. Global, Regional, and National Estimates of Rotavirus Mortality in Children <5 Years of Age, 2000–2013. *Clin. Infect. Dis.* **2016**, *62* (Suppl. S2), S96–S105. [CrossRef] [PubMed]
5. Sadiq, A.; Khan, J. Rotavirus in developing countries: Molecular diversity, epidemiological insights, and strategies for effective vaccination. *Front. Microbiol.* **2023**, *14*, 1297269. [CrossRef] [PubMed]
6. Burnett, E.; Parashar, U.D.; Tate, J.E. Real-world effectiveness of rotavirus vaccines, 2006–2019: A literature review and meta-analysis. *Lancet Glob. Health* **2020**, *8*, e1195–e1202. [CrossRef]
7. Desselberger, U. Differences of Rotavirus Vaccine Effectiveness by Country: Likely Causes and Contributing Factors. *Pathogens* **2017**, *6*, 65. [CrossRef]
8. Parker, E.P.; Ramani, S.; Lopman, B.A.; Church, J.A.; Iturriza-Gomara, M.; Prendergast, A.J.; Grassly, N.C. Causes of impaired oral vaccine efficacy in developing countries. *Future Microbiol.* **2018**, *13*, 97–118. [CrossRef]
9. Desselberger, U. Rotaviruses. *Virus Res.* **2014**, *190*, 75–96. [CrossRef]
10. Matthijnssens, J.; Otto, P.H.; Ciarlet, M.; Desselberger, U.; Van Ranst, M.; Johne, R. VP6-sequence-based cutoff values as a criterion for rotavirus species demarcation. *Arch. Virol.* **2012**, *157*, 1177–1182. [CrossRef]
11. Matthijnssens, J.; Ciarlet, M.; McDonald, S.M.; Attoui, H.; Banyai, K.; Brister, J.R.; Buesa, J.; Esona, M.D.; Estes, M.K.; Gentsch, J.R.; et al. Uniformity of rotavirus strain nomenclature proposed by the Rotavirus Classification Working Group (RCWG). *Arch. Virol.* **2011**, *156*, 1397–1413. [CrossRef] [PubMed]
12. RCWG. 2023. Available online: https://rega.kuleuven.be/cev/viralmetagenomics/virus-classification/rcwg (accessed on 15 March 2025).
13. Sadiq, A.; Bostan, N.; Jadoon, K.; Aziz, A. Effect of rotavirus genetic diversity on vaccine impact. *Rev. Med. Virol.* **2022**, *32*, e2259. [CrossRef] [PubMed]
14. Doro, R.; Farkas, S.L.; Martella, V.; Banyai, K. Zoonotic transmission of rotavirus: Surveillance and control. *Expert Rev. Anti Infect. Ther.* **2015**, *13*, 1337–1350. [CrossRef] [PubMed]
15. Bányai, K.; Pitzer, V.E. Chapter 2.10—Molecular Epidemiology and Evolution of Rotaviruses. In *Viral Gastroenteritis*; Svensson, L., Desselberger, U., Greenberg, H.B., Estes, M.K., Eds.; Academic Press: Boston, MA, USA, 2016; pp. 279–299.
16. Bányai, K.; Gentsch, J. Special issue on 'Genetic diversity and evolution of rotavirus strains: Possible impact of global immunization programs'. *Infect. Genet. Evol.* **2014**, *28*, 375–376. [CrossRef]
17. Vita, D.; Lemos, M.; Neto, Z.; Evans, M.; Francisco, N.M.; Fortes, F.; Fernandes, E.; Cunha, C.; Istrate, C. High Detection Rate of Rotavirus Infection Among Children Admitted with Acute Gastroenteritis to Six Public Hospitals in Luanda Province After the Introduction of Rotarix((R)) Vaccine: A Cross-Sectional Study. *Viruses* **2024**, *16*, 1949. [CrossRef]
18. Gentsch, J.R.; Glass, R.I.; Woods, P.; Gouvea, V.; Gorziglia, M.; Flores, J.; Das, B.K.; Bhan, M.K. Identification of group A rotavirus gene 4 types by polymerase chain reaction. *J. Clin. Microbiol.* **1992**, *30*, 1365–1373. [CrossRef]
19. Iturriza-Gomara, M.; Kang, G.; Gray, J. Rotavirus genotyping: Keeping up with an evolving population of human rotaviruses. *J. Clin. Virol.* **2004**, *31*, 259–265. [CrossRef]
20. Hall, T.A. BioEdit: A user-friendly biological sequence alignement editor and analysis program for windows 95/98/NT. *Nucleic Acids Symp.* **1999**, *41*, 95–98.
21. Larkin, M.A.; Blackshields, G.; Brown, N.P.; Chenna, R.; McGettigan, P.A.; McWilliam, H.; Valentin, F.; Wallace, I.M.; Wilm, A.; Lopez, R.; et al. Clustal W and Clustal X version 2.0. *Bioinformatics* **2007**, *23*, 2947–2948. [CrossRef]
22. Nicholas, K.B.; Nicholas, H.B.; Deerfield, D.W. GeneDoc: Analysis and visualization of genetic variation. *EMBnet News* **1997**, *4*, 1–4.
23. Kumar, S.; Stecher, G.; Tamura, K. MEGA7: Molecular Evolutionary Genetics Analysis Version 7.0 for Bigger Datasets. *Mol. Biol. Evol.* **2016**, *33*, 1870–1874. [CrossRef] [PubMed]

24. Felsenstein, J. Evolutionary trees from DNA sequences: A maximum likelihood approach. *J. Mol. Evol.* **1981**, *17*, 368–376. [CrossRef]
25. Aoki, S.T.; Settembre, E.C.; Trask, S.D.; Greenberg, H.B.; Harrison, S.C.; Dormitzer, P.R. Structure of Rotavirus Outer-Layer Protein VP7 Bound with a Neutralizing Fab. *Science* **2009**, *324*, 1444–1447. [CrossRef] [PubMed]
26. Dormitzer, P.R.; Nason, E.B.; Prasad, B.V.; Harrison, S.C. Structural rearrangements in the membrane penetration protein of a non-enveloped virus. *Nature* **2004**, *430*, 1053–1058. [CrossRef] [PubMed]
27. Dormitzer, P.R.; Sun, Z.Y.; Wagner, G.; Harrison, S.C. The rhesus rotavirus VP4 sialic acid binding domain has a galectin fold with a novel carbohydrate binding site. *EMBO J.* **2002**, *21*, 885–897. [CrossRef]
28. Zeller, M.; Patton, J.T.; Heylen, E.; Coster, S.D.; Ciarlet, M.; Ranst, M.V.; Matthijnssens, J. Genetic Analyses Reveal Differences in the VP7 and VP4 Antigenic Epitopes between Human Rotaviruses Circulating in Belgium and Rotaviruses in Rotarix and RotaTeq. *J. Clin. Microbiol.* **2012**, *50*, 966–976. [CrossRef]
29. Esteves, A.; Nordgren, J.; Pereira, J.; Fortes, F.; Dimbu, R.; Saraiva, N.; Mendes, C.; Istrate, C. Molecular epidemiology of rotavirus in four provinces of Angola before vaccine introduction. *J. Med. Virol.* **2016**, *88*, 1511–1520. [CrossRef] [PubMed]
30. Omatola, C.A.; Ogunsakin, R.E.; Olaniran, A.O. Prevalence, Pattern and Genetic Diversity of Rotaviruses among Children under 5 Years of Age with Acute Gastroenteritis in South Africa: A Systematic Review and Meta-Analysis. *Viruses* **2021**, *13*, 1905. [CrossRef]
31. Bawa, F.K.; Mutocheluh, M.; Dassah, S.D.; Ansah, P.; Oduro, A.R. Genetic diversity of rotavirus infection among young children with diarrhoea in the Kassena-Nankana Districts of Northern Ghana: A seasonal cross-sectional survey. *Pan Afr. Med. J.* **2023**, *44*, 148. [CrossRef]
32. Munlela, B.; Joao, E.D.; Strydom, A.; Bauhofer, A.F.L.; Chissaque, A.; Chilaule, J.J.; Mauricio, I.L.; Donato, C.M.; O'Neill, H.G.; de Deus, N. Whole-Genome Characterization of Rotavirus G9P[6] and G9P[4] Strains That Emerged after Rotavirus Vaccine Introduction in Mozambique. *Viruses* **2024**, *16*, 1140. [CrossRef]
33. Gasparinho, C.; Piedade, J.; Mirante, M.C.; Mendes, C.; Mayer, C.; Vaz Nery, S.; Brito, M.; Istrate, C. Characterization of rotavirus infection in children with acute gastroenteritis in Bengo province, Northwestern Angola, prior to vaccine introduction. *PLoS ONE* **2017**, *12*, e0176046. [CrossRef] [PubMed]
34. Bonura, F.; Mangiaracina, L.; Filizzolo, C.; Bonura, C.; Martella, V.; Ciarlet, M.; Giammanco, G.M.; De Grazia, S. Impact of Vaccination on Rotavirus Genotype Diversity: A Nearly Two-Decade-Long Epidemiological Study before and after Rotavirus Vaccine Introduction in Sicily, Italy. *Pathogens* **2022**, *11*, 424. [CrossRef] [PubMed]
35. Joao, E.D.; Munlela, B.; Chissaque, A.; Chilaule, J.; Langa, J.; Augusto, O.; Boene, S.S.; Anapakala, E.; Sambo, J.; Guimaraes, E.; et al. Molecular Epidemiology of Rotavirus A Strains Pre- and Post-Vaccine (Rotarix®) Introduction in Mozambique, 2012–2019: Emergence of Genotypes G3P[4] and G3P[8]. *Pathogens* **2020**, *9*, 671. [CrossRef] [PubMed]
36. Mhango, C.; Banda, A.; Chinyama, E.; Mandolo, J.J.; Kumwenda, O.; Malamba-Banda, C.; Barnes, K.G.; Kumwenda, B.; Jambo, K.C.; Donato, C.M.; et al. Comparative whole genome analysis reveals re-emergence of human Wa-like and DS-1-like G3 rotaviruses after Rotarix vaccine introduction in Malawi. *Virus Evol.* **2023**, *9*, vead030. [CrossRef]
37. Seheri, L.M.; Magagula, N.B.; Peenze, I.; Rakau, K.; Ndadza, A.; Mwenda, J.M.; Weldegebriel, G.; Steele, A.D.; Mphahlele, M.J. Rotavirus strain diversity in Eastern and Southern African countries before and after vaccine introduction. *Vaccine* **2018**, *36*, 7222–7230. [CrossRef]
38. Ramachandran, M.; Das, B.K.; Vij, A.; Kumar, R.; Bhambal, S.S.; Kesari, N.; Rawat, H.; Bahl, L.; Thakur, S.; Woods, P.A.; et al. Unusual diversity of human rotavirus G and P genotypes in India. *J. Clin. Microbiol.* **1996**, *34*, 436–439. [CrossRef]
39. Page, N.A.; Seheri, L.M.; Groome, M.J.; Moyes, J.; Walaza, S.; Mphahlele, J.; Kahn, K.; Kapongo, C.N.; Zar, H.J.; Tempia, S.; et al. Temporal association of rotavirus vaccination and genotype circulation in South Africa: Observations from 2002 to 2014. *Vaccine* **2018**, *36*, 7231–7237. [CrossRef]
40. Gurgel, R.Q.; Cuevas, L.E.; Vieira, S.C.; Barros, V.C.; Fontes, P.B.; Salustino, E.F.; Nakagomi, O.; Nakagomi, T.; Dove, W.; Cunliffe, N.; et al. Predominance of rotavirus P[4]G2 in a vaccinated population, Brazil. *Emerg. Infect. Dis.* **2007**, *13*, 1571–1573. [CrossRef]

viruses

MDPI

Article

Unveiling the Genomic Landscape of G2P[6] Rotavirus a Strains in Brazil: Evolutionary and Epidemiological Perspectives

Vanessa Cristina Martins Silva [1,2], Yasmin França [1,2], Lais Sampaio de Azevedo [1,2], Raquel Guiducci [1], Edlaine Faria de Moura Villela [2] and Adriana Luchs [1,2,*]

1 Virology Center, Adolfo Lutz Institute, Sao Paulo 01246-902, Brazil
2 Graduate Program in Sciences of the Center for Disease Control, São Paulo State Department of Health, Sao Paulo 01246-000, Brazil
* Correspondence: driluchs@gmail.com or adriana.luchs@ial.sp.gov.br; Tel.: +55-11-3068-2984

Abstract

In Brazil, molecular surveillance expanded after Rotarix™ vaccine introduction, alongside G2P[4] dominance. The G2P[6] genotype, despite sharing the same DS-1-like constellation as G2P[4] strains, remains rare. This retrospective study analyzed eight Brazilian G2P[6] strains (2012–2014) through RT-PCR and 11-segments sequencing, followed by phylogenetic analysis. Two distinct groups were identified: 2012–2013 strains (six) carried a DS-1-like backbone with the rare NSP4 E6 genotype, while 2014 strains (two) exhibited the classical DS-1-like constellation with E2. Phylogenetic analysis confirmed the two main clusters: 2012–2013 strains related to classical G2P[4] and uncommon global genotypes, and 2014 strains resembling emerging DS-1-like G1/G3/G8P[8] reassortants. The 2012–2013 strains clustered within G2-VP7 Lineage IVa, while the 2014 strains belonged to Lineage V, reflecting the global distribution of these variants. All VP4 genes were classified within the P[6]-Ia lineage, with phylogenetic analyses suggesting separate introductions from Asia and Africa. The E6 NSP4 gene segment identified in these strains has an undetermined origin and was not previously associated with G2P[6] strains in Brazil. Despite similarities to G2P[4], G2P[6] strains remain rare, with no genomic features explaining their limited spread. Phylogenetic data indicate multiple reassortment events and international viral exchange, highlighting Brazil's role in RVA diversity. Ongoing full-genome surveillance is crucial to track rare variants and assess their public health relevance.

Keywords: molecular surveillance; gastroenteritis; Genetic diversity; rotavirus; public health

1. Introduction

Rotavirus alphagastroenteritidis (https://ictv.global/ accessed on 4 July 2025), also known as Rotavirus A (RVA), is a major cause of acute diarrhea in young children worldwide and also affects a broad spectrum of animal species [1,2]. It belongs to the genus *Rotavirus*, within the subfamily *Sedoreoviridae*, the family *Reovirales*, and the realm *Riboviria* [3]. Its genome consists of eleven segments of double-stranded RNA (dsRNA), encoding six structural proteins (VP1–VP4, VP6 and VP7) and five or six non-structural proteins (NSP1–NSP5/6) [4]. Traditionally, RVA strains were classified using a binary system based on the outer capsid proteins VP7 and VP4, referred to as G and P genotypes, respectively [5]. The genotypes G1P[8], G2P[4], G3P[8], G4P[8], G9P[8] and G12P[8] represent the six most prevalent strains found in humans [5,6].

https://doi.org/10.3390/v17081103

To enable a more comprehensive genomic characterization, the RVA classification system was expanded to include all 11 genome segments, with the current nomenclature assigning specific genotypes to each segment: Gx–P[x]–Ix–Rx–Cx–Mx–Ax–Nx–Tx–Ex–Hx [7,8]. Most human RVA strains fall into one of three major genome constellations: the Wa-like genogroup 1 (Gx–P[x]–I1–R1–C1–M1–A1–N1–T1–E1–H1), the DS-1-like genogroup 2 (Gx–P[x]–I2–R2–C2–M2–A2–N2–T2–E2–H2) and, less commonly, the AU-1-like genogroup 3 (Gx–P[x]–I3–R3–C3–M3–A3–N3–T3–E3–H3) [7,8]. Following the introduction of the RVA genome constellation classification, whole-genome analyses of all 11 gene segments have revealed the virus's genetic diversity, shaped by point mutations, gene rearrangements, inter- and intra-species reassortment and, to a lesser extent, homologous recombination [7,9].

Brazil has been conducting a genotypic surveillance of RVA strains for several decades, with efforts significantly intensified after the introduction of the Rotarix™ vaccine into the national immunization program in 2006 [6,10–14]. Afterward this implementation, a marked increase in the detection of the G2P[4] genotype was observed [6,15–17]. This phenomenon, of global significance, was also reported in multiple countries subsequent to the launch of universal RVA vaccination and initially led to the hypothesis that it might be associated with vaccine-driven selective pressure [18–22]. However, studies conducted thereafter, including those in countries without RVA vaccine coverage, suggest that more complex mechanisms related to viral ecology may be involved [23–27]. Between 2007 and 2010, the G2P[4] predominated throughout Latin America and the Caribbean, underscoring its high dissemination capacity [28].

In contrast, the G2P[6] genotype did not emerge widely in either vaccinated or non-vaccinated regions, remaining rare in human populations, despite sharing a DS-1-like backbone genotype constellation resembling that of G2P[4] [6,14,29–36]. This genotype exhibited an uneven pattern of emergence, being detected at low frequencies in various parts of the world, including Sub-Saharan Africa, Asia and Latin America [6,14,29,31,34,35,37]. Studies indicate that different lineages of the P[6] genotype may have originated from multiple interspecies reassortment events involving RVA from different animal hosts, accounting for the significant genetic heterogeneity observed in this genotype [38–40]. This association with zoonotic events and its predominance in neonatal infections reinforce the complexity of its transmission dynamics, a trend that has also been documented in Brazil [41–45].

The number of available full genome sequences for G2P[6] remains limited, largely due to its low prevalence [33,35]. To better understand the factors that limit the selective advantage of G2P[6] compared to G2P[4], it is essential to perform a complete genome sequencing of these strains in order to identify potential selective pressures influencing their spread. The aim of this study was to perform a molecular characterization and phylogenetic analysis of the 11 genome segments of eight Brazilian G2P[6] RVA strains identified between 2007 and 2014, to enhance understanding of the complex transmission dynamics and evolutionary fitness of this rare genotype. The findings are expected to contribute to a better understanding of viral ecology and support improved surveillance efforts in Brazil and beyond.

2. Material and Methods

2.1. Study Design and Sample Selection

This retrospective study analyzed convenience fecal samples from individuals of all age groups, collected through Brazil's national viral gastroenteritis surveillance program, between 2007 and 2014. Sample processing was carried out at the Enteric Diseases Center

(NDE) of the Adolfo Lutz Institute (IAL), a macro-regional reference center responsible for monitoring viral gastroenteritis in the Midwest and parts of the Southeast and South regions, under the coordination of the Ministry of Health (MS). For this study, all samples that tested positive for the G2P[6] genotype during routine surveillance at IAL were selected for further analysis. Specifically, eight G2P[6] strains were included: five strains identified in 2012 [6], one in 2013 and two in 2014 [34], originating from the states of São Paulo (Southeast region) and Paraná (South region) (Table 1).

Table 1. Demographic and spatial data, migration profile of dsRNA segments, genotype constellation and lineages of RVA G2P[6] strains, Brazil, 2007–2014. The rare genotype E6-NSP4 and common genotype E2-NSP4 are highlighted in lilac.

Strain	Age	Gender	City	State	Profile	VP7	VP4	VP6	VP1	VP2	VP3	NSP1	NSP2	NSP3	NSP4	NSP5
						G2	P[6]	I2	R2	C2	M2	A2	N2	T2	E6	H2
RVA/Human-wt/BRA/IAL-R1000/2012/G2P[6]	2 months	F	São Paulo	SP	Short	IVa	I-a	V	V	IVa	V	IVa	V	V	-	IVa
RVA/Human-wt/BRA/IAL-R1007/2012/G2P[6]	4 months	F	São Paulo	SP	Short	IVa	I-a	V	V	IVa	V	IVa	V	V	-	IVa
RVA/Human-wt/BRA/IAL-R1142/2012/G2P[6]	2 months	M	São Paulo	SP	Short	IVa	I-a	V	V	IVa	V	IVa	V	V	-	IVa
RVA/Human-wt/BRA/IAL-R1175/2012/G2P[6]	1 year	F	São Paulo	SP	Short	IVa	I-a	V	V	IVa	V	-	V	V	-	IVa
RVA/Human-wt/BRA/IAL-R1228/2012/G2P[6]	10 months	M	Nova Laran-jeiras	PR	Short	IVa	I-a	V	V	IVa	V	IVa	V	V	-	IVa
RVA/Human-wt/BRA/IAL-R126/2013/G2P[6]	4 years	F	São Paulo	SP	Short	IVa	I-a	V	V	IVa	V	IVa	V	V	-	IVa
Strain	**Age**	**Gender**	**City**	**State**	**Profile**	**VP7**	**VP4**	**VP6**	**VP1**	**VP2**	**VP3**	**NSP1**	**NSP2**	**NSP3**	**NSP4**	**NSP5**
						G2	P[6]	I2	R2	C2	M2	A2	N2	T2	E2	H2
RVA/Human-wt/BRA/IAL-R50/2014/G2P[6]	26 days	U	São Paulo	SP	Short	V	I-a	V	V	IVa	V	IVa	V	V	VI	IVa
RVA/Human-wt/BRA/IAL-R52/2014/G2P[6]	22 days	M	São Paulo	SP	Short	V	I-a	V	V	IVa	V	IVa	V	V	VI	IVa

SP: São Paulo state; PR: Paraná state; M: male; F: female; U: unidentified.

2.2. *Electropherotyping Analysis*

RVA migration patterns were assessed by polyacrylamide gel electrophoresis (PAGE), followed by silver staining for visualization, as described by Herring et al. (1982) [46].

2.3. *Whole-Genome Constellation Profiling*

RVA dsRNA was extracted from 10% fecal suspensions using the Quick-DNA/RNA™ Viral MagBead Kit (Zymo Research®, Orange, CA, USA), according to the manufacturer's instructions. RT-PCRs targeting the 11 genome segments were performed in-house using the following published primers: NSP1 [47–49]; NSP2, NSP4 and VP6 [48,49]; NSP3 and NSP5/6 [49]; VP1, VP2 and VP3 [50]; VP4 [51]; and VP7 [49,52]. Amplification conditions followed the protocol described by Gouvea et al. (1990) [52].

PCR products were resolved on 1.5% agarose gels stained with GelRed™ (Biotium, Fremont, CA, USA), alongside a 100 bp molecular-size ladder, and visualized using a gel documentation system. Amplicons were subsequently sequenced using the BigDye™ Terminator v3.1 Cycle Sequencing Kit (Applied Biosystems, Foster City, CA, USA), with the same primers used for PCR. Sequencing was carried out on an ABI 3500 Genetic Analyzer (Applied Biosystems) at the Premium Network of Multi-User Equipment/IMT/FMUSP.

Chromatograms were manually edited using Sequencher™ 4.7 software (Gene Codes Corporation, Ann Arbor, MI, USA). Genotype assignment was performed using the Rotavirus A Genotyping Tool v0.1 (https://mpf.rivm.nl/mpf/typingtool/rotavirusa/ accessed on 1 November 2024).

2.4. Phylogenetic Inference

Sequences obtained in this study were aligned with reference RVA sequences for the genes NSP1–NSP5/6 and VP1–VP4, VP6 and VP7 retrieved from GenBank. Alignments were performed using the CLUSTAL W algorithm implemented in BioEdit v7.0.5.2 (Ibis Therapeutics, Carlsbad, CA, USA). Maximum likelihood (ML) phylogenetic trees were constructed for each gene segment using MEGA X [53], and the best-fitting nucleotide substitution models were selected according to the corrected Akaike Information Criterion (AICc). The following models were applied: T92+G+I for NSP1 (A2), VP1 (R2), VP3 (M2) and VP7 (G2); GTR+G+I for NSP2 (N2), T92+G for NSP3 (T2), NSP4 (E2) and NSP5 (H2); T92+I for NSP4 (E6); TN93+G for VP2 (C2); and HKY+G+I for VP4 (P[6]) and VP6 (I2). Branch support was assessed with 1000 bootstrap replicates.

Reference strains were included for lineage assignment based on previously published studies: Agbemabiese et al. (2019) [54] and Azevedo et al. (2023) [55] for DS-1-like constellations, Gupta et al. (2021) [56] for VP4 P[6] and Doan et al. (2015) [57] for VP7. Pairwise nucleotide identity was calculated using distance matrices in MEGA X [53].

3. Results

3.1. Genome Constellations

The G2P[6] RVA strains exhibited the characteristic short electropherotype associated with P[6] genotypes. Near-complete nucleotide sequences were obtained for the NSP1–NSP5/6, VP7 and VP6 segments, and partial sequences for the VP1–VP4 genes of eight G2P[6] strains. An exception was strain IAL-R1175/2012, for which only a partial NSP1 sequence could be obtained. The percentage of the genome sequenced among the strains ranged from 47.4% to 59.2%. The sequence lengths and the nucleotide positions analyzed for the eight G2P[6] strains are detailed in Table S1.

The two G2P[6] strains detected in 2014 (IAL-R50 and IAL-R52) exhibited the classical DS-1-like genomic constellation (I2-R2-C2-M2-A2-N2-T2-E2-H2), while the five strains from 2012 (IAL-R1000, IAL-R1007, IAL-R1142, IAL-R1175 and IAL-R1228) and the single strain from 2013 (IAL-R126) presented a DS-1-like backbone associated with the rare E6 genotype in the NSP4 segment (I2-R2-C2-M2-A2-N2-T2-E6-H2) (Table 1).

3.2. Analysis of the Outer Capsid Glycoprotein VP7

Globally representative strains from the five known G2 lineages (I, II, III, IVa, IVnon-a and V) were included in this analysis. The Brazilian G2P[6] strains analyzed in this study clustered separately. Strains IAL-R1007/2012, IAL-R1000/2012, IAL-R1228/2012, IAL-R1142/2012, IAL-R1175/2012 and IAL-R126/2013 grouped within Lineage IVa, exhibiting nucleotide identities ranging from 99.9% to 100%. In contrast, strains IAL-R52/2014 and IAL-R50/2014 were classified within Lineage V, sharing 99.5% nucleotide identity with each other (Table 1, Figure 1A).

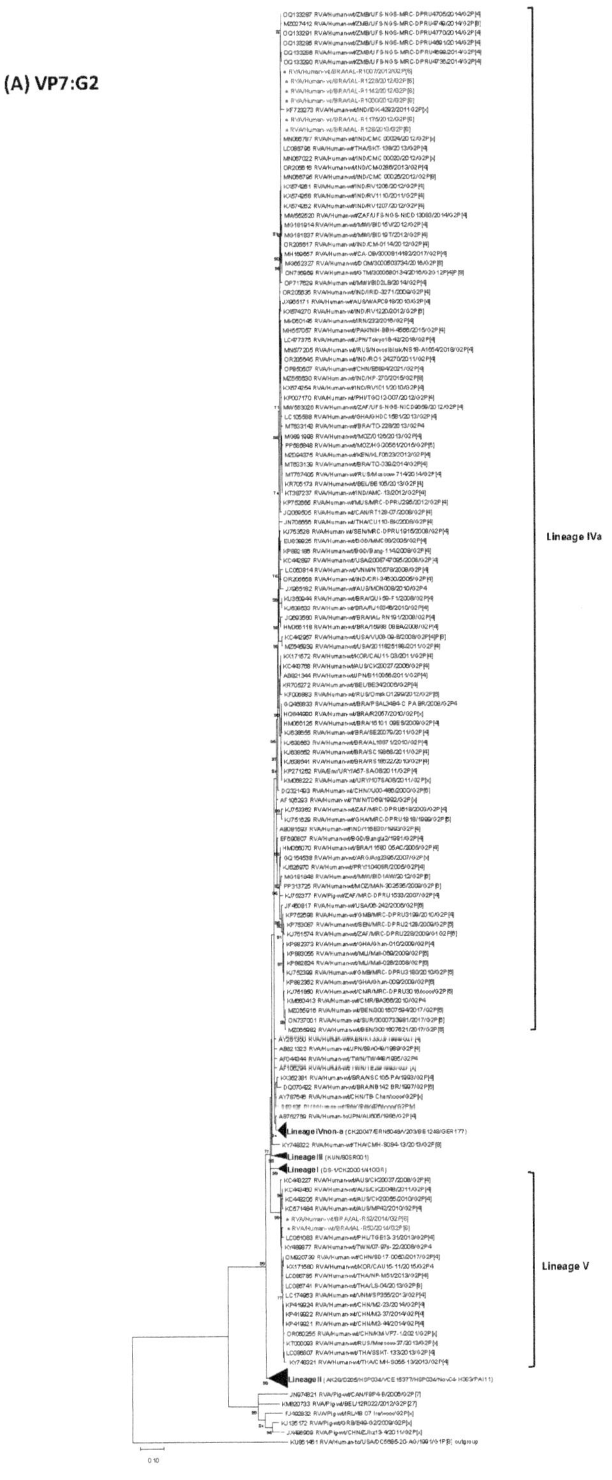

Figure 1. *Cont.*

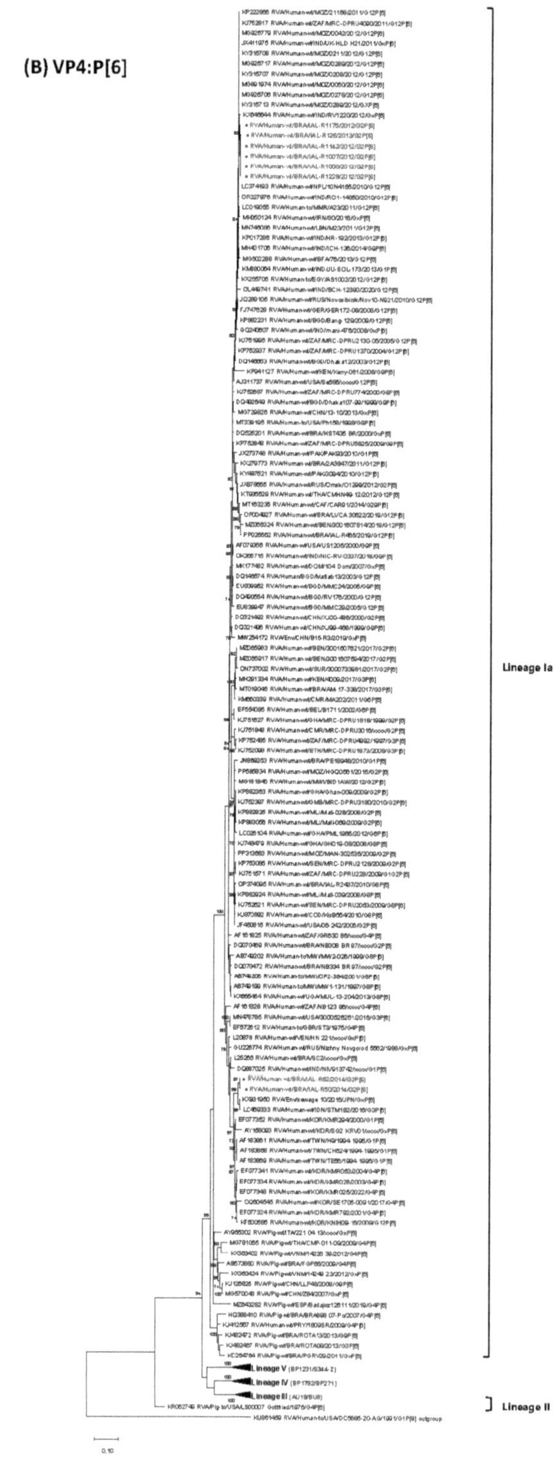

Figure 1. *Cont.*

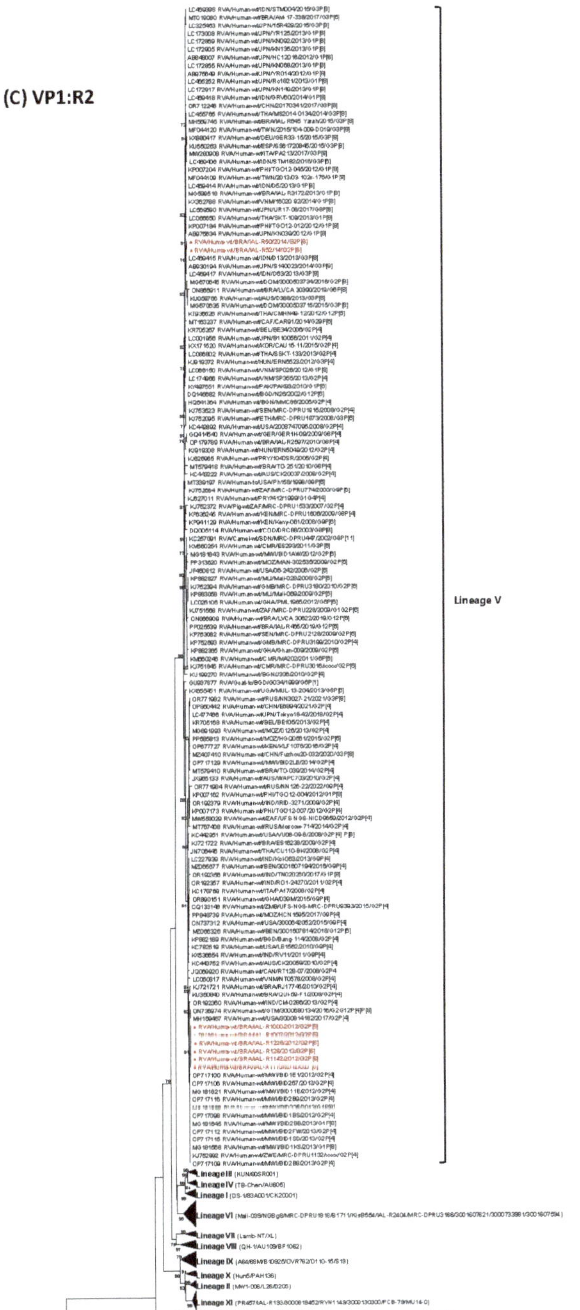

Figure 1. *Cont.*

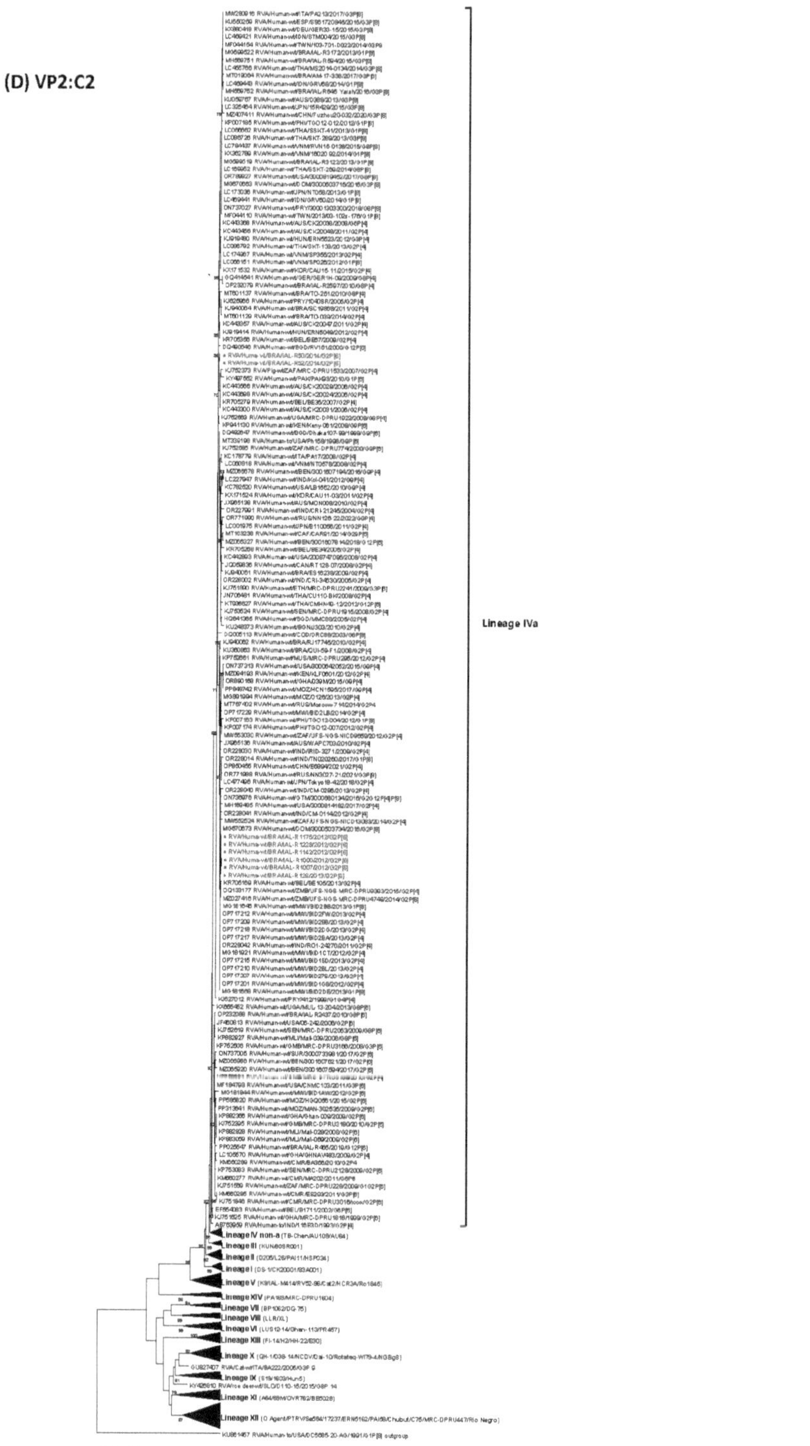

Figure 1. *Cont.*

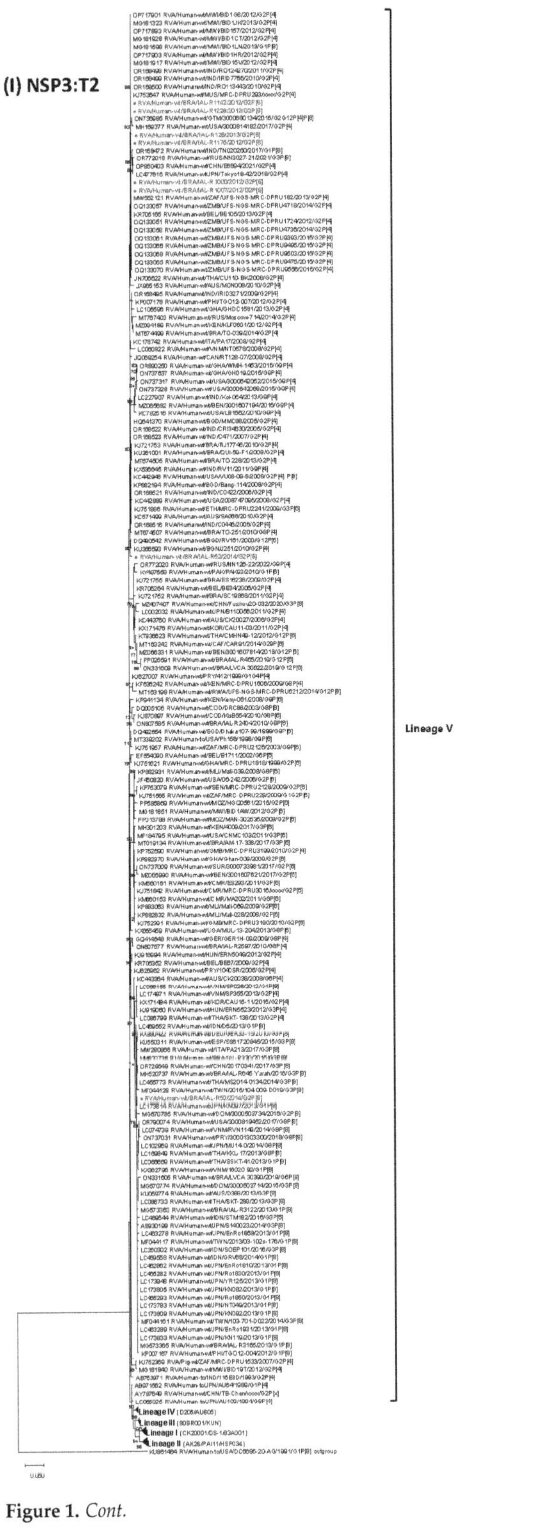

Figure 1. *Cont.*

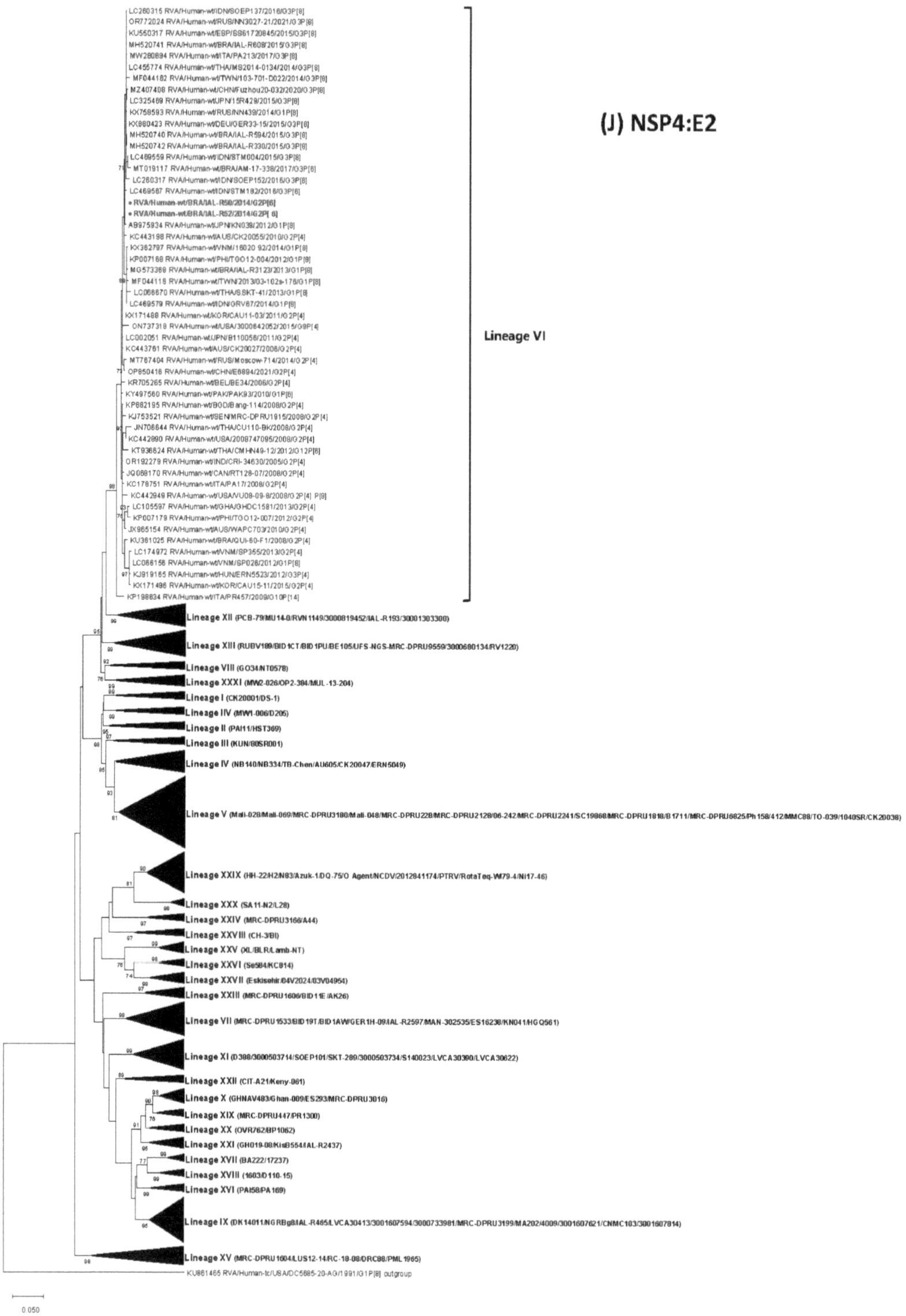

Figure 1. *Cont.*

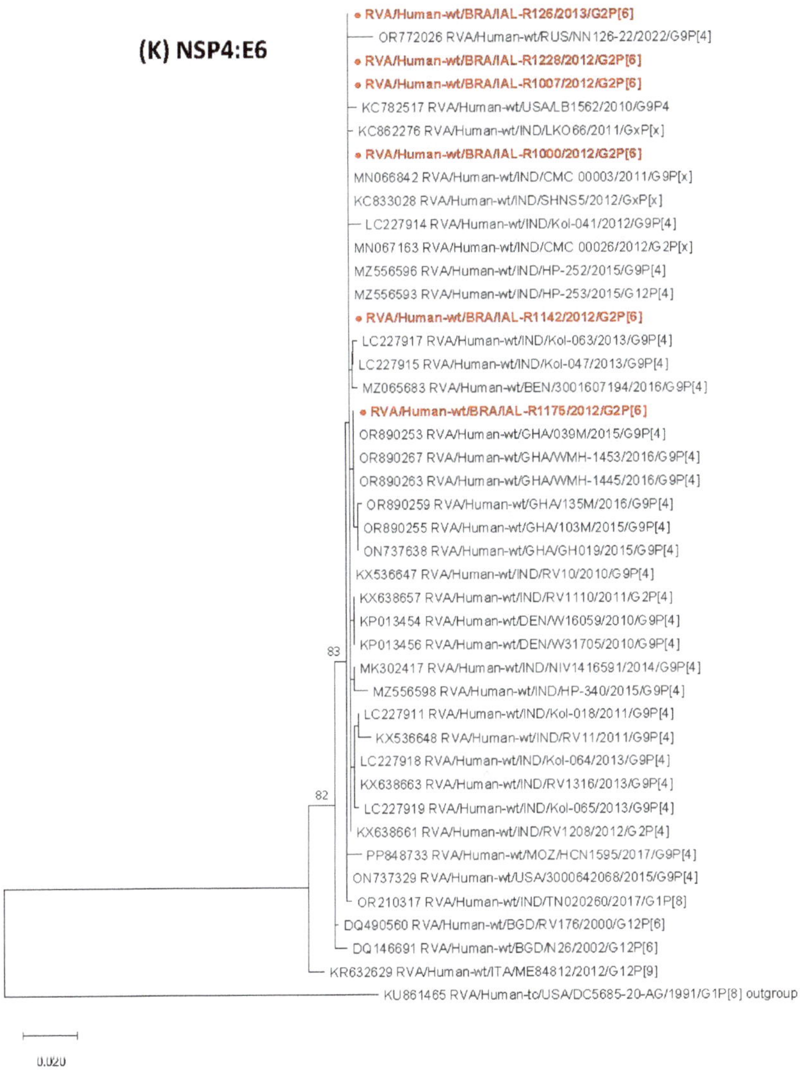

Figure 1. *Cont.*

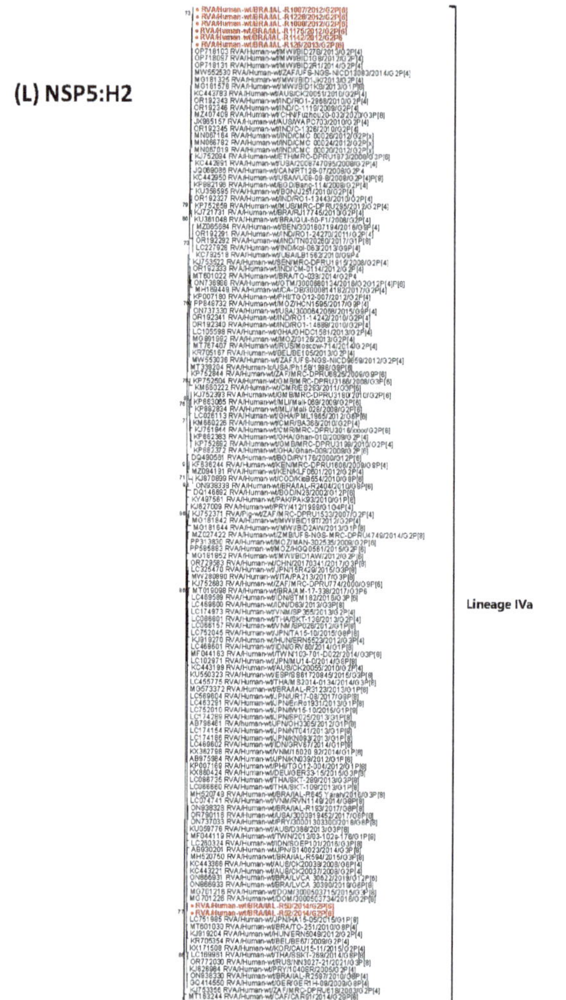

Figure 1. Maximum likelihood phylogenetic trees based on nucleotide sequences of 11 genome segments [VP7-G2 (**A**), VP4-P[6] (**B**), VP1-R2 (**C**), VP2-C2 (**D**), VP3-M2 (**E**), VP6-I2 (**F**), NSP1-A2 (**G**), NSP2-N2 (**H**), NSP3-T2 (**I**), NSP4-E2 (**J**), NSP4-E6 (**K**) and NSP5/6-H2 (**L**)] were constructed using MEGA X software to assess the genetic relatedness of eight Brazilian G2P[6] RVA strains (IAL-R1007/2012, IAL-R1000/2012, IAL-R1228/2012, IAL-R1142/2012, IAL-R1175/2012, IAL-R126/2013, IAL-R52/2014 and IAL-R50/2014; shown in bold red) to global reference strains, with bootstrap values indicated at nodes and scale bars representing nucleotide substitutions per site.

Strains from Lineage IVa (IAL-R1007/2012, IAL-R1000/2012, IAL-R1228/2012, IAL-R1142/2012, IAL-R1175/2012 and IAL-R126/2013) exhibited a high nucleotide identity (99.0–100%) with classical G2P[4]/G2P[x] strains detected between 2009 and 2017 in geographically diverse areas, including India, Thailand, Australia, Zambia, Malawi, South Africa, the United States, Pakistan, Ireland and Mauritius. They also demonstrated close similarity (99.2–99.8% nt) to atypical genotypes, such as G2G12P[4]P[8] and G2P[8], reported in India, Zambia, the Dominican Republic and Guatemala between 2012 and 2016. Conversely, these Lineage IVa strains were more distantly related to earlier Brazilian G2P[4]/G2P[x] strains identified across the country, such as 11580_05AC/2005 (95.6–95.9% nt), IAL-RN191/2008 (96.6–96.9% nt), 15988_08BA/2008 (97.5–97.9% nt), QUI-59-F1/2008 (97.2–97.5% nt), PSAL3484-C_PA_BR/2008 (97.1–97.3% nt), 16101_09ES/2009 (97.1–97.4% nt), AL18871/2010 (97.4–97.6% nt), R2057/2010 (97.2% nt), RJ18346/2010 (96.9–97.3% nt), RS18622/2010 (97.1–97.4% nt), SE20079/2011 (97.3–97.5% nt), SC19868/2011 (97.1–97.4% nt), TO-228/2013 (98.2–98.8% nt) and TO-039/2014 (98.4–98.6% nt) (Figure 1A).

Strains IAL-R52/2014 and IAL-R50/2014 (Lineage V) were closely related to G2P[4]/G2P[x] strains detected between 2008 and 2021 in Taiwan, Australia, Thailand, China, South Korea, Vietnam, Russia and the Philippines, showing nucleotide identities of 98.2–99.3%. They also shared 99.1% nt identity with the atypical strain RVA/Human-wt/THA/LS-04/2013/G2P[8]. The RVA/Human-wt/BRA/NB142/1997/G2P[6] strain, identified in hospitalized neonates with community-acquired diarrhea during a G2P[6] outbreak in Belém, Pará, in 1997 [28,42], did not share a lineage with any of the Brazilian strains described herein (88–92.7% nt) (Figure 1A).

3.3. Analysis of the Spike Protein VP4

Regarding the VP4 gene, all eight Brazilian G2P[6] strains analyzed in this study clustered within Lineage P[6]-Ia, occupying two different branches. Strains IAL-R1000/2012, IAL-R1007/2012, IAL-R1142/2012, IAL-R1228/2012, IAL-R1175/2012 and IAL-R126/2013 exhibited high nucleotide identity (99.0–99.6%) with atypical G12P[6]/GxP[6]/G9P[6] strains detected in Africa (Mozambique; South Africa) and Asia (Myanmar; Nepal; India). On the other hand, strains IAL-R50/2014 and IAL-R52/2014 were genetically closer to Asian strains exclusively, encompassing RVA/Env/sewage_10/2016/JPN/GxP[6] (98.5–98.8% nt) and RVA/Human-wt/IDN/STM182/2016/G3P[6] (98.1–98.4% nt) (Table 1, Figure 1B).

Compared to previously reported Brazilian P[6] RVA strains, IAL-R1000/2012, IAL-R1007/2012, IAL-R1142/2012, IAL-R1228/2012, IAL-R1175/2012, IAL R126/2013, IAL-R50/2014 and IAL-R52/2014 displayed greater genetic divergence, with lower nucleotide identities when aligned with HST435_BR/2000/GxP[6] (92.5–96.9% nt), 2A3847/2011/G12P[6] (90.7–95.6% nt), LVCA_30622/2019/G12P[6] (89.2–94.3% nt), IAL-R465/2019/G12P[6] (89.5–94.9% nt), AM-17-338/2017/G3P[6] (90.5–94% nt), PE18948/2010/G1P[6] (91.7–94.3% nt), IAL-R2437/2010/G8P[6] (91.2–94.8% nt) and SC2/xxxx/GxP[6] (92.7–95.8% nt). This divergence also extended to strains identified in neonatal patients from Belém, comprising RVA/Human-wt/BRA/NB334/1997/G2P[6] and RVA/Human-wt/BRA/NB308/1997/G2P[6] (92.3–97% nt) [42]. Moreover, the Brazilian IAL P[6] strains showed significant genetic differences from swine-origin P[6] strains (84.4–89.6% nt), including those previously reported in Brazil (84.5–89.5% nt) (Figure 1B).

3.4. Phylogenetic Analysis of VP1–VP3 and VP6

Phylogenetic analyses of the VP1, VP2, VP3 and VP6 gene segments revealed that the Brazilian strains IAL-R1000/2012, IAL-R1007/2012, IAL-R1142/2012, IAL-R1228/2012,

IAL-R1175/2012 and IAL-R126/2013 clustered closely together, sharing high nucleotide identity (≥99.3 nt). These strains formed a distinct phylogenetic branch separate from the other two Brazilian G2P[6] RVA strains, IAL-R50/2014 and IAL-R52/2014, which also exhibited high mutual similarity (≥99.8% nt). Despite clustering separately, all strains were classified within the same lineages: R2-V, C2-IVa, M2-V and I2-V (Table 1, Figure 1C–F).

Comparative analysis revealed that the Brazilian strains IAL-R1000/2012, IAL-R1007/2012, IAL-R1142/2012, IAL-R1228/2012, IAL-R1175/2012 and IAL-R126/2013 exhibited significant nucleotide sequence similarity (≥99% nt) in the VP1, VP2 and VP3 gene segments when compared with classical G2P[4] strains possessing a DS-1-like genomic constellation reported worldwide between 2005 and 2021. These reference strains were broadly distributed across Africa, Europe, the Americas, Asia and Oceania (South Africa; Kenya; Mauritius; Mozambique; Malawi; Zambia; Zimbabwe; Belgium; Russia; USA; Canada; India; Bangladesh; China; Japan; Australia). Furthermore, the same Brazilian G2P[6] strains demonstrated notable genetic similarity (99–99.8% nt) in the VP1 and VP2 segments with atypical strains, including G9P[4], G12P[4]P[8], G2G12P[4]P[8] and G2P[8], identified from 2010 to 2017 in Mozambique, USA, India, Benin, Guatemala and the Dominican Republic. In addition, a high nucleotide identity (≥99% nt) in VP1, VP2 and VP3 genes was also observed between the Brazilian G2P[6] IAL-R1000/2012, IAL-R1007/2012, IAL-R1142/2012, IAL-R1228/2012, IAL-R1175/2012 and IAL-R126/2013 strains and emergent double-reassortant G1P[8] DS-1-like strains found in Malawi and the Philippines during 2012–2013 (Figure 1C–E).

The Brazilian G2P[6] strains IAL-R50/2014 and IAL-R52/2014 exhibited elevated nucleotide similarity in the VP1, VP2 and VP3 genes with emerging double-reassortant strains, including G1P[8] DS-1-like, equine-like G3P[8] DS-1-like and bovine-like G8P[8] DS-1-like genotypes detected worldwide, notably in Latin America and Asia. Specifically, the VP1 gene showed 99.0–99.5% nt identity with strains circulating between 2012 and 2017 in Asian countries (Japan; India; the Philippines; China; Taiwan; Vietnam; Thailand), as well as 99.1–99.2% nt identity with a Brazilian G1P[8] DS-1-like strain from 2013 (IAL-R3172; MG599518) (Figure 1C). Likewise, the VP2 gene exhibited 99.0–99.2% nt similarity with double-reassortant strains circulating from 2012 to 2018 in India, Thailand, Paraguay, USA, the Dominican Republic, Japan, Vietnam and Australia, in addition to 99.0% nt identity with the Brazilian G1P[8] DS-1-like (IAL-R3122; MG599519) and equine-like G3P[8] DS-1-like (IAL-R645_Yarah; MH569752) strains detected in 2013 and 2016, respectively. Furthermore, the VP2 gene also showed close relation (99.0–99.4% nt) to the G2P[4] and uncommon G8P[4]/G6P[4]/G9P[6]/G1G4P[4]/G3P[4] strains documented between 1999 and 2015 across Australia, Asia, Europe and Africa (Figure 1D). The VP3 gene also shared high identity (99.0–99.5% nt) with double-reassortant strains detected globally from 2013 through 2021 (Australia; India; the Czech Republic; Japan; Thailand; China; Taiwan; Vietnam; USA; the Dominican Republic; Germany; Spain; Russia; Paraguay), and 99.0–99.4% nt similarity with Brazilian G1P[8] DS-1-like (IAL-R3123; MG599524), equine-like G3P[8] DS-1-like (IAL-R645_Yarah; MH569758) and bovine-like G8P[8] DS-1-like (IAL-R193; OP407951) strains isolated from 2013 to 2017 (Figure 1E).

Finally, analysis of the VP6 gene revealed a binary clustering pattern among the Brazilian G2P[6] strains, dividing them into two distinct branches [strains 2012–2013 versus strains 2014] consistent with the distribution previously observed for other genomic segments (VP1–VP4 and VP7). The 2012–2013 strains exhibited high nucleotide identity (≥99.0% nt) with a broad range of classical G2P[4]/G2P[x] strains (2006–2018), atypical G2G12P[4]P[8]/G9P[4]/G12P[4]/G3P[6]/G12P[6] genotypes (1997–2017), including the RVA/Human-wt/RUS/O1299/2012/G2P[6] (99.2–99,4% nt), and emerging double-reassortant G1P[8] DS-1-like/equine-like G3P[8] DS-1-like strains (2013–2020) from

Asia, Africa, Europe and the Americas. Similarly, the 2014 strains shared high similarity (99.1–99.8% nt) with double-reassortant G1P[8] DS-1-like and equine-like G3P[8] DS-1-like strains circulating between 2012 and 2017 across multiple regions, including Brazil (RVA/Human-wt/BRA/IAL-R3123/2013/G1P[8]; RVA/Human-wt/BRA/IAL-R645_Yarah/2016/G3P[8]) (99.4–99.8% nt). Despite this divergence, both clusters showed close nucleotide identity with a shared set of reference strains, including classical G2P[4] strains detected in Bangladesh and Senegal in 2008 and 2010, respectively (99.0–99.6% nt), as well as unusual strains, such as G3P[4] and G2P[4]P[8], recognized during the 2008–2012 period in Hungary and the USA (99.0–99.4% nt) (Figure 1F).

3.5. Phylogenetic Analysis of NSP1-NSP5 Genes

Consistent with the pattern observed for the structural proteins VP1–VP3 and VP6, phylogenetic analyses of the non-structural proteins NSP1, NSP2 and NSP5 likewise displayed a binary clustering trend. The Brazilian G2P[6] strains IAL-R1000/2012, IAL-R1007/2012, IAL-R1142/2012, IAL-R1228/2012, IAL-R1175/2012 and IAL-R126/2013 clustered together, exhibiting a nucleotide identity ranging from 99.0% to 100%, whereas strains IAL-R50/2014 and IAL-R52/2014 grouped separately (≥99.1% nt among them) (Figure 1G,H,L). On the other hand, the NSP3 and NSP4 gene segments exhibited a distinct genetic landscape, with NSP4 shifting from genotype E6 (2012–2013 strains) to E2 (2014 strains) (Figure 1I–K).

Phylogenetic analysis of the NSP1 gene revealed that Brazilian G2P[6] strains from 2012 to 2013 [placed in Lineage R2-IVa] clustered together and showed high nucleotide identity (99.0–99.9% nt) with traditional G2P[4] strains detected worldwide (2005–2015), G2P[4] strains documented in Brazil in 2008–2010 (99–99.3% nt), and several uncommon genotypes identified across Asia, Africa and the Americas over the decades (1997–2018) (99–99.6%nt). They were also closely related to emergent DS-1-like double-reassortant strains (G1P[8]; equine-like G3P[8]; bovine-like G8P[8]) reported globally between 2012 and 2018 (99–99.3% nt), including Brazilian representatives (RVA/Human-wt/BRA/IAL-R3122/2013/G1P[8]; RVA/Human-wt/BRA/LVCA_30390/2019/G6P[8]; RVA/Human-wt/BRA/IAL-R193/2017/G8P[8]) (99.0–99.2% nt). Conversely, the IAL 2014 G2P[6] strains [classified within Lineage R2-IVa] showed similarity in NSP1 with classical G2P[4] strains from Australia and Belgium, detected in 2006, and non-classical G12P[6]/G3P[4] strains reported in Thailand in 2012, Hungary in 2012 and Brazil in 2019 [LVCA_30413; ON331602] (99–99.3% nt). As expected, these strains were genetically related to G1P[8]/G6P[8]/G8P[8] DS-1-like reassortant strains identified in Vietnam (RVA/Human-wt/VNM/SP026/2012/G1P[8]) and Brazil (RVA/Human-wt/BRA/LVCA_30390/2019/G6P[8]; RVA/Human-wt/BRA/IAL-R193/2017/G8P[8]) (99–99.1% nt). Both clusters shared high nucleotide identity (99–99.9% nt) with a common set of reference strains from diverse genotypes and regions, including G2P[4] (AUS 2006, BEL 2006), G12P[6] (THA 2012, BRA 2019), G1P[8] DS-1-like (VNM 2012), G3P[4] (HUN 2012), G6P[8] and G8P[8] (BRA 2017–2019) (Table 1, Figure 1G). The IAL-R1175/12 strain was excluded from the NSP1 segment analyses due to its very short sequence, which was interfering with the alignments and phylogenetic inferences.

In relation to the NSP2 gene, strains IAL-R1000/2012, IAL-R1007/2012, IAL-R1142/2012, IAL-R1228/2012, IAL-R1175/2012 and IAL-R126/2013 [grouped within Lineage N2-V] showed high nucleotide identity (≥99.2% nt) with traditional G2P[4] strains from India, Malawi and Zambia (2012–2015), and with unusual G2P[8]/G9P[4] strains from Zambia, USA and India (2008–2014) (≥99.3% nt). They also shared similarity (99.6–99.9% nt) with double-reassortant G1P[8] DS-1-like strains from Malawi (2013). Strains IAL-R50/2014 and IAL-R52/2014 [assigned to Lineage N2-V] exhibited 99.0–99.4% nt identity with

G2P[4] strains from Italy, Belgium, South Korea and Brazil (2006–2011). These strains also showed genetic relationship (99.0–99.1% nt) to atypical G2P[8] and G3P[6] genotypes from India and the Dominican Republic (2016), and with double-reassortant G1P[8] DS1-like and equine-like G3P[8] DS1-like strains (99.0–99.7% nt) recognized internationally (2012–2015), including Brazilian strains from 2013 (IAL-R3123/G1P[8]) and 2016 (IAL-R645_Yarah/G3P[8]) (99.0–99.4% nt) (Table 1, Figure 1H).

As for the NSP3 gene, phylogenetic analysis indicated that strains IAL from 2012–2013, belonging to Lineage T2-V (≥99% nt among them), formed a well-supported cluster with standard G2P[4] strains circulating between 2005 and 2021 in Africa, Asia, Oceania, Europe and North America continents (≥99.0% nt), and were also homologous to Brazilian G2P[4] strains from 2008–2014 (99.0–99.5% nt). These strains further showed high similarity (99.0–99.7% nt) to atypical genotypes (G2P[8]; G3P[6]; G12P[6]; G9P[4]; G2G12P[4]P[8]) identified in the USA, Ethiopia, Bangladesh, India and Guatemala (2000–2016), aligned with strain RVA/Human-wt/BRA/TO-251/2010/G8P[4] (99.0–99.1% nt), and were related to G1P[8] DS-1-like and equine-like G3P[8] DS-1-like strains from India (2017) and Russia (2021) (99.1–99.5% nt). Brazilian IAL 2014 strains clustered separately from each other (shared 98.3% nt identity). Strain IAL-R52/2014 [Lineage T2-V] grouped with G2P[4] strains from 1999–2011 in Mauritius, India, Bangladesh, Australia, Italy, USA and Brazil (2008–2013) (99.0–99.3% nt), and was also similar (9.2–99.3% nt) to non-classical genotypes (G2P[4]P[8]; G3P[6]; G12P[6]; G1G4P[4]) reported during 1999–2009 in the USA, Ethiopia, Bangladesh, Paraguay and Brazil (RVA/Human-wt/BRA/TO-251/2010/G8P[4]) (99.0% nt). Meanwhile, strain IAL-R50/2014 [Lineage T2-V] clustered exclusively with G2P[4] strains from Asia (2013–2015) (99.0–99.2% nt), and showed 99.1–99.3% nt similarity with non-classical G6P[4]/G3P[4]/G2P[8]/G3P[6] strains circulating in Australia, Hungary, the Dominican Republic and India (2008–2016). It also exhibited high identity (99.0–99.8% nt) with emergent double-reassortant G1P[8]/G3P[8]/G8P[8] strains detected globally (2012–2017), including Brazilian strains IAL-R3122/2013/G1P[8], IAL-R3165/2013/G1P[8] and IAL-R330/2015/G3P[8] (99.2–99.6% nt). In the NSP3 gene, a high nucleotide identity (99–100%) was also observed between the IAL 2012–2013 and 2014 strains, which shared a common set of global reference strains, including G2P[4] strains from Mauritius, India (2005–2007, 2011), the USA (2008), Bangladesh (2005, 2008), Australia (2010), Italy (2008) and Brazil (2008–2013); G3P[6] from Ethiopia (2009); G8P[4] from Brazil (2010); G9P[4] from India (2011); and G12P[6] from Bangladesh (2000) (Table 1, Figure 1I).

The Brazilian strains IAL-R50/2014 and IAL-R52/2014, classified within the NSP4 E2-VI lineage, exhibited elevated nucleotide similarity (99.0–99.9% nt) with a wide range of classical (G2P[4]), atypical (G1P[6]; G3P[6]) and double-reassortant (G1P[8] DS-1-like; equine-like G3P[8] DS-1-like) strains detected across the globe between 2005 and 2021, including previously reported Brazilian strains (RVA/Human-wt/BRA/IAL-R594/2015/G3P[8]; RVA/Human-wt/BRA/IAL-R608/2015/G3P[8]; RVA/Human-wt/BRA/IAL-R330/2015/G3P[8]; RVA/Human-wt/BRA/IAL-R3123/2013/G1P[8]; RVA/Human-wt/BRA/AM-17-338/2017/G3P[6]) (99.1–99.9% nt). These IAL 2014 E2-VI strains exhibited 100% nt identity among themselves and clustered distinctly from the G2P[6] strains linked to the 1997 neonates' outbreak from Belém [42], which belong to Lineage IV [NB334; NB140] (Table 1, Figure 1J). Strains IAL-R1000/2012, IAL-R1007/2012, IAL-R1142/2012, IAL-R1228/ 2012, IAL-R1175/2012 and IAL-R126/2013 (≥99.8% nt between them) are members of the rare NSP4 E6 genotype, for which no lineages have been defined so far, and exhibited high nucleotide identity with classical G2P[4]/G2P[x] strains (≥99.7% nt) from India (2011–2012), as well as with uncommon or not-typed G9P[4]/G9P[x]/G[x]P[x]/G12P[4]/G12P[6] strains (≥99.% nt) from India, Ghana, USA,

Denmark, Bangladesh, Mozambique, Russia and Benin (2000–2022). Among the strains showing 100% nucleotide identity, the most notable include G9P[4] strains from India (2010–2015), Ghana (2015–2016) and the USA (2010), as well as G2P[x] (2012), G9P[x] (2011), GxP[x] (2012), G12P[4] (2015) and G2P[4] strains (2012), with all of them identified in India (Table 1, Figure 1K).

Lastly, NSP5 gene analysis revealed that strains IAL-R1000/2012, IAL-R1007/2012, IAL-R1142/2012, IAL-R1228/2012, IAL-R1175/2012 and IAL-R126/2013 exhibited high nucleotide identity (99.0–99.8%) with typical G2P[4] strains widespread across Africa, Asia, the Americas and Oceania from 2008 to 2014. They also displayed significant similarity (99.2–99.6% nt) with Brazilian G2P[4] strains (2008–2014) and atypical G9P[4]/G2P[4]P[8]/G3P[6]/G2G12P[4]P[8] genotypes identified in Mozambique, the USA, Ethiopia and Guatemala (2008–2017). Moreover, these strains clustered with emerging double-reassortant DS-1-like G1P[8] and equine-like G3P[8] DS-1-like strains from Malawi and China (2013–2020), with nucleotide identity ranging from 99.5% to 99.8%. Strains IAL-R50/2014 and IAL-R52/2014 showed high nucleotide identity (99.2–99.6%) with classical G2P[4] strains from 2003–2015 across Paraguay, South Africa, Europe, Asia and Australia. They were also closely related (99.0–99.6% nt) to diverse atypical genotypes (G6P[6]; G6P[4]; G1G4P[4]; G2P[8]; G8P[4]; G3P[4]; G29P[6]; G3P[6]; G9P[6]) reported between 1999 and 2016 worldwide and highly similar (99.1–99.8% nt) to unusual Brazilian strains (G8P[4]; G12P[6]; G6P[8]; G3P[6]) from 2010 to 2019. Furthermore, these strains clustered with emerging double-reassortant G1P[8]/G3P[8]/G8P[8] strains circulating globally from 2012 to 2021, including Brazilian isolates (RVA/Human-wt/BRA/IAL-R3123/2013/G1P[8]; RVA/Human-wt/BRA/IAL-R594/2015/G3P[8]; RVA/Human-wt/BRA/IAL-R645_Yarah/2016/G3P[8]; RVA/Human-wt/BRA/IAL-R193/2017/G8P[8]) (99.0–99.8% nt) (Table 1, Figure 1L).

Interestingly, the IAL 2014 NSP5 strains exhibited high nucleotide similarity to G2P[6] strains detected in the USA in 2006 [06-242] (99–99.1% nt), as well as in the African continent in 1999 [GHA/MRC-DPRU1818], 2009 [SEN/MRC-DPRU2128; MOZ/MAN-302535] and 2015 [MOZ/HGQ0561] (99–99.3% nt). They also showed close similarity to the mixed RVA/Human-wt/ZAF/MRC-DPRU228/2009/G1G2P[6] strain (99.0–99.1% nt). Notably, both groups of strains (IAL 2012–2013 and IAL 2014) showed high similarity with the RVA/Human-tc/USA/Ph158/1998/G9P[6] strain, with nucleotide identities of 99.2–99.4% for the 2014 strains and 99.0–99.1% nt for the 2012–2013 strains. A comparable pattern was observed in the VP6, NSP1 and NSP3 genes, reinforcing the genetic consistency across these segments (Figure 1L).

4. Discussion

This study provides a comprehensive 11-segments analysis of eight G2P[6] RVA strains identified in Brazil between 2007 and 2014. Given the limited availability of sequencing data for RVA G2P[6] strains [33,42,58–60], the findings herein provide valuable insights into the genomic diversity and evolutionary dynamics of this uncommon genotype, particularly regarding strains of American origin.

Phylogenetic reconstructions exposed the existence of two genetically distinct clusters: strains from 2012–2013 displaying I2-R2-C2-M2-A2-N2-T2-E6-H2 constellation, and strains from 2014 exhibiting a pure DS-1-like genomic backbone (I2-R2-C2-M2-A2-N2-T2-E2-H2). The vast majority of G2P[6] strains deposited in GenBank are associated with the conserved DS-1-like constellation (I2-R2-C2-M2-A2-N2-T2-E2-H2), predominantly of African origin [58–60], with only a single representative strain from the Americas (RVA/Human-wt/USA/06-242/2006/G2P[6]) having all 11 genomic segments sequenced [33]. This same genetic backbone was also observed in the Brazilian 2014 strains characterized in this study (IAL-R50 and IAL-R52), further supporting this common association.

On the other hand, the Brazilian 2012–2013 strains exhibited the rare E6 genotype (I2-R2-C2-M2-A2-N2-T2-E6-H2), which, to date, has not been reported in association with the G2P[6] genotype. The uncommon E6 genotype was first identified in a human G8P[6] strain in India in 2000 and was subsequently detected in G12P[6] strains in Bangladesh (2000–2001) and in a G12P[9] strain in Italy (2012) [61–63]. Studies suggest a possible animal origin for the E6 genotype [62,64]. The I2-R2-C2-M2-A2-N2-T2-E6-H2 genomic constellation appears to be more frequently linked to the G9P[4] genotype, as reported in several regions, including Latin America [35,65–67]. It has been proposed that this constellation emerged through multiple reassortment events involving DS-1-like strains and other strains donating the NSP4 segment (E6) [66]. Similar reassortment events may have occurred between the Brazilian G2P[6] strains identified in 2012–2013 and other co-circulating strains. However, the phylogenetic analyses conducted in this study were unable to confirm such events, likely due to the limited availability of full-genome sequences from Brazilian strains, particularly atypical G9P[4] genotypes. These findings underscore the need to expand the full-genome sequencing of RVA strains in Brazil, especially for rare or unusual genotypes [68–70]. Interestingly, G9P[4]-E6 strains, which were frequently detected between 2009 and 2016, declined after 2017, and the E6 genotype has not been reported since [64]. Recent data from Iran (2021–2022) and the Czech Republic (2018) indicate the replacement of E6 by E2 in G9P[4] strains [71,72]. Extrapolating this trend to our genetic findings, it is plausible that a similar replacement occurred in the Brazilian IAL G2P[6] strains detected in 2014, which also presented the NSP4-E2 genotype instead of E6.

The G2 VP7 gene evolved through successive lineage replacements, reflecting genetic changes and possible reassortment events over time, with its evolutionary history indicating diversification into five major lineages (I–V) [57,73,74]. G2 strains were initially dominated by Lineages I–III and gradually replaced by Lineage IVnon-a between 1985 and 1996. From 1999 onward, a clear shift toward Lineage IVa occurred, which has remained globally dominant since the early 2000s [57,73,74]. Although G2-IVnon-a variants are less common, both sub-lineages have been reported to co-circulate, suggesting concurrent transmission in some regions [21,75,76]. Lineage V emerged around 2005–2006 and now predominates among modern G2 strains [77]. Interestingly, its antigenic profile is similar to G2-IVnon-a strains, suggesting that its emergence was likely due to intragenotypic reassortment rather than antigenic escape [57]. A phylogenetic analysis of eight Brazilian IAL G2P[6] strains showed that six (IAL-R1000/2012, IAL-R1007/2012, IAL-R1142/2012, IAL-R1228/2012, IAL-R1175/2012 and IAL-R126/2013) clustered within Lineage IVa, while strains IAL-R50/2014 and IAL-R52/2014 belonged to VP7 G2 Lineage V. These findings align with the global evolutionary pattern of the G2 VP7 gene, indicating coexistence and possible transition between these lineages in the Brazilian context as well.

Phylogenetic analysis of the VP4 gene in Brazilian G2P[6] strains revealed their affiliation with the P[6]-Ia lineage, alongside globally circulating human genotypes such as G12P[6], G1P[6], G9P[6], G8P[6], G4P[6], G3P[6] and G6P[6] [70,78–81]. The P[6]-Ia lineage also includes porcine and porcine-like human strains reported worldwide [39,82,83]; nevertheless, the IAL strains examined in this study showed no evidence of zoonotic origin. Additionally, the Brazilian IAL P[6] strains segregated into two clusters: those from 2012–2013 grouped with African and Asian strains, while the 2014 strains clustered exclusively with Asian lineages. This phylogenetic pattern reflects the complex geographic spread and epidemiological dynamics of the P[6]-Ia lineage. Compared to earlier Brazilian P[6] RVA strains, the sequences analyzed here exhibited greater genetic divergence [42,70,84,85], indicating likely independent introductions into Brazil, possibly from Africa and Asia.

This also suggests gaps in local surveillance, which may have impaired the detection of previously circulating Brazilian strains.

Considering VP7 and VP4 together, further functional studies focusing on amino acid variations involved in antigenicity and host interactions, given their demonstrated roles in modulating viral fitness, immune evasion, and transmissibility through changes in antigenic epitopes and host cell binding, could provide additional insights into potential differences in these viral properties [36,69,70,73].

Phylogenetic analyses of the 11 gene segments of Brazilian G2P[6] strains revealed the presence of two temporally and genetically distinct groups. Group 1, comprising strains detected between 2012 and 2013 (IAL-R1000/2012, R1007/2012, R1142/2012, R1228/2012, R1175/2012, and R126/2013), showed high internal similarity and was clearly divergent from Group 2, represented by the 2014 strains (IAL-R50/2014 and IAL-R52/2014), which also clustered separately, with high nucleotide identity between them.

Group 1 (strains 2012–2013) clustered with globally distributed classical G2P[4] strains circulating between 2005 and 2021 [21,36,86,87]. The IAL G2P[6] 2012–2013 strains were strongly related to earlier Brazilian G2P[4] strains (2008–2014) [88,89], as well as to atypical genotypes such as G9P[4], G3P[4] and G12P[6] identified across multiple continents [65,66,84,90]. They also showed similarities to DS-1-like double-reassortant strains, including equine-like G3P[8], G1P[8] and G8P[8] strains circulating in Africa, Asia, Europa, North America and Latin America, including Brazil, between 2012 and 2021 [59,69,91,92]. Notably, they harbored the rare NSP4 E6 genotype, which has been associated with emergent strains in distinct geographic contexts and showed high nucleotide identity with strains from Asia and Africa [64,93]. The genetic similarities with strains from diverse continents highlight the existence of a highly dynamic and interconnected global viral pool, marked by the circulation of both human and potentially zoonotic lineages, positioning Brazil as a potential hotspot for genetic reassortment and recombination.

Group 2 (strains 2014) appeared to be associated with emergent DS-1-like genetic constellations. The presence of the NSP4 E2-IV lineage, frequently found in recently emerging DS-1-like G1P[8] and equine-like G3P[8] strains, supports this hypothesis [94–96]. The IAL G2P[6] 2014 strains were clearly genetically related to emergent DS-1-like double-reassortant strains, predominantly detected in Asia, as well as to previously reported Brazilian strains [96–99]. In addition, although to a lesser extent than their similarity with emergent DS-1-like strains, they also exhibited relatedness to classical G2P[4] strains and atypical genotypes such as G9P[4] and G3P[6] [58,85,86,90,97]. Their robust genetic similarity to Brazilian DS-1-like double-reassortant strains identified in 2013 and 2016 [96,99] suggests that the IAL G2P[6] 2014 strains were rapidly integrated into the local viral landscape. This finding highlights the adaptability of emergent DS-1-like strains and their ability to establish themselves in new epidemiological settings through reassortment with locally circulating strains, underscoring 2014 as a pivotal year in the local diversification of G2P[6] variants.

Furthermore, the lack of phylogenetic continuity between the studied Brazilian G2P[6] strains and previously reported strains from Brazil, North America or Africa [33,42,59,60] reinforces the hypothesis of multiple independent introduction events into Brazil, likely through distinct routes involving Africa, Asia and Latin America. The consistent binary clustering pattern observed across multiple structural and non-structural gene segments indicates that the observed diversity results from both viral migration and local reassortment events involving international and regional lineages. This highlights the dynamic interplay between viral dispersal and genome plasticity in shaping the local viral population.

A noteworthy point is that the DS-1-like constellation identified in the IAL G2P[6] strains shows a strong genetic connection with emerging intergenogroup DS-1-like human strains, such as G1/G3/G8P[8], reported globally, including in Brazil [59,69,91,92,96–99].

In contrast, the rare G12P[6] DS-1-like strains detected during 2011–2020 and recently analyzed at the full-genome level in Brazil [70], show no genetic evidence of relatedness to these emergent intergenogroup DS-1-like strains. The distinct evolutionary trajectories observed for the two P[6]-bearing strains, G2P[6] and G12P[6], despite their sharing nearly identical DS-1-like genomic backbones, underscore the complex interplay of selective pressures shaping RVA evolution. Although both strains circulate under similar ecological conditions in Brazil and contribute minimally to the RVA-associated diarrheal disease burden, with limited detection rates, factors beyond genomic constellation, such as host immunity, viral fitness and ecological competition, play a critical role in determining their persistence and dissemination.

5. Conclusions

In conclusion, the Brazilian G2P[6] strains analyzed in this study reflect a complex evolutionary and epidemiological dynamic, originating from multiple genetic sources and showing links to both classical and emerging strains. These findings reveal a scenario characterized by multiple reassortment events and extensive international circulation, underscoring the highly dynamic nature of the G2P[6] genotype and its strong potential for evolution. The genetic relatedness to strains from diverse geographic regions suggests that factors such as population mobility, international trade, and migration flows have influenced the introduction and spread of these strains in Brazil. No clear genomic or phylogenetic differences explaining why G2P[4] holds greater epidemiological importance compared to G2P[6] could be identified. Both genotypes share DS-1-like constellations, exhibit multiple introductions of distinct RVA strains into the human population, and display genetic diversification. It was not possible to pinpoint a specific genetic or evolutionary factor underlying the higher epidemiological relevance of G2P[4] in diarrheal disease. Collectively, these data emphasize the importance of ongoing molecular surveillance of RVA diversity, particularly focusing on variants with potential epidemiological impact.

Supplementary Materials: The following supporting information can be downloaded at: https://www.mdpi.com/article/10.3390/v17081103/s1. Table S1: Length and nucleotide position of each gene segment of the Brazilian RVA G2P[6] strains detected in Brazil, 2007–2014.

Author Contributions: Conceptualization, A.L.; methodology, V.C.M.S., Y.F., L.S.d.A., R.G., E.F.d.M.V. and A.L.; formal analysis, V.C.M.S., Y.F., L.S.d.A. and A.L.; data curation, V.C.M.S., L.S.d.A. and R.G.; writing—original draft preparation, V.C.M.S. and A.L.; writing—review and editing, Y.F., L.S.d.A., R.G. and E.F.d.M.V.; supervision, E.F.d.M.V. and A.L.; project administration, A.L.; funding acquisition, E.F.d.M.V. and A.L. All authors have read and agreed to the published version of the manuscript.

Funding: This study was funded by the Sao Paulo Research Foundation (FAPESP) through grant numbers #2020/14786-0 to Adriana Luchs and #2021/09064-8 to Yasmin França. The National Council for Scientific and Technological Development is a government agency under the Ministry of Science and Technology of the Brazilian federal government (CNPq) #310056/2023-3 to Adriana Luchs. Special Health Fund for Mass Immunization and Disease Control (Fundo Especial de Saúde para Imunização em Massa e Controle de Doenças-FESIMA) CAF Nº #017/2023 and #042/2024 to Adriana Luchs. Graduate Support Program—Financial Support for Educational or Research Projects (Programa de Apoio à Pós-Graduação-Auxílio Financeiro a Projeto Educacional ou de Pesquisa-PROAP-AUXPE) #2022/115 to Vanessa Cristina Martins Silva, Lais Sampaio de Azevedo and Yasmin França. Coordination for the Improvement of Higher Education Personnel—Scholarship and Support (Management System Coordenação de Aperfeiçoamento de Pessoal de Nível Superior-Sistema de Controle de Bolsas e Auxílio-CAPES-SCBA) #2022-0/88881.689557 to Lais Sampaio de Azevedo.

Institutional Review Board Statement: Ethical approval was granted by the Adolfo Lutz Institute, São Paulo, Brazil, on 10 March 2015 (protocol number CAAE 40718114.5.0000.0059) and on

11 November 2021 (protocol number CAAE 51963821.3.0000.0059). Study participants were not required to provide informed consent because the Ethics Committee classified this study as part of routine surveillance activities.

Data Availability Statement: Nucleotide sequences from this study were submitted to GenBank with accession numbers: NSP1: PV126468–PV126475; NSP2: PV126476–PV126483; NSP3: PV126484–PV126491; NSP4: PV299264–PV299271; NSP5: PV335520–PV335527; VP1: PV299272–PV299279; VP2: PV335407–PV335414; VP3: PV335415–PV335422; VP4: PV335423–PV335430; VP6: PV335644–PV335651; and VP7: PV335652–PV335659.

Conflicts of Interest: The authors declare no conflict of interest.

References

1. Šenica, P.; Žele Vengušt, D.; Vengušt, G.; Kuhar, U. Genomic revelations: Investigating rotavirus a presence in wild ruminants and its zoonotic potential. *Front. Vet. Sci.* **2024**, *11*, 1429654. [CrossRef] [PubMed]
2. Prunas, O.; Asare, E.O.; Sajewski, E.; Li, Y.; Pithawala, Z.; Weinberger, D.M.; Warren, J.L.; Armah, G.E.; Cunliffe, N.A.; Iturriza-Gómara, M.; et al. Global estimates of rotavirus vaccine efficacy and effectiveness: A rapid review and meta-regression analysis. *EClinicalMedicine* **2025**, *81*, 103122. [CrossRef] [PubMed]
3. Matthijnssens, J.; Attoui, H.; Bányai, K.; Brussaard, C.P.D.; Danthi, P.; Del Vas, M.; Dermody, T.S.; Duncan, R.; Fang, Q.; Johne, R.; et al. ICTV Virus Taxonomy Profile: Sedoreoviridae 2022. *J. Gen. Virol.* **2022**, *103*, e001782. [CrossRef] [PubMed]
4. Esona, M.D.; Steele, D.; Kerin, T.; Armah, G.; Peenze, I.; Geyer, A.; Page, N.; Nyangao, J.; Agbaya, V.A.; Trabelsi, A.; et al. Determination of the G and P types of previously nontypeable rotavirus strains from the African Rotavirus Network, 1996–2004: Identification of unusual G types. *J. Infect. Dis.* **2010**, *202* (Suppl. S1), S49–S54. [CrossRef]
5. Amin, A.B.; Cates, J.E.; Liu, Z.; Wu, J.; Ali, I.; Rodriguez, A.; Panjwani, J.; Tate, J.E.; Lopman, B.A.; Parashar, U.D. Rotavirus Genotypes in the Postvaccine Era: A Systematic Review and Meta-analysis of Global, Regional, and Temporal Trends by Rotavirus Vaccine Introduction. *J. Infect. Dis.* **2024**, *229*, 1460–1469. [CrossRef]
6. Luchs, A.; Cilli, A.; Morillo, S.G.; Carmona, R.d.C.; Timenetsky, M.d.C.S.T. Rotavirus genotypes circulating in Brazil, 2007–2012: Implications for the vaccine program. *Rev. Inst. Med. Trop. Sao Paulo* **2015**, *57*, 305–313. [CrossRef]
7. Díaz Alarcón, R.G.; Salvatierra, K.; Gómez Quintero, E.; Liotta, D.J.; Parreño, V.; Miño, S.O. Complete Genome Classification System of *Rotavirus alphagastroenteritidis*: An Updated Analysis. *Viruses* **2025**, *17*, 211. [CrossRef]
8. Matthijnssens, J.; Ciarlet, M.; McDonald, S.M.; Attoui, H.; Bányai, K.; Brister, J.R.; Buesa, J.; Esona, M.D.; Estes, M.K.; Gentsch, J.R.; et al. Uniformity of rotavirus strain nomenclature proposed by the Rotavirus Classification Working Group (RCWG). *Arch. Virol.* **2011**, *156*, 1397–1413. [CrossRef]
9. Hoxie, I.; Dennehy, J.J. Intragenic recombination influences rotavirus diversity and evolution. *Virus Evol.* **2020**, *6*, vez059. [CrossRef]
10. Santos, N.; Soares, C.C.; Volotão, E.M.; Albuquerque, M.C.M.; Hoshino, Y. Surveillance of rotavirus strains in Rio de Janeiro, Brazil, from 1997 to 1999. *J. Clin. Microbiol.* **2003**, *41*, 3399–3402. [CrossRef]
11. Leite, J.P.G.; Carvalho-Costa, F.A.; Linhares, A.C. Group A rotavirus genotypes and the ongoing Brazilian experience: A review. *Mem. Inst. Oswaldo Cruz* **2008**, *103*, 745–753. [CrossRef] [PubMed]
12. da Silva Soares, L.; de Fátima Dos Santos Guerra, S.; do Socorro Lima de Oliveira, A.; da Silva Dos Santos, F.; de Fátima Costa de Menezes, E.M.; Mascarenhas, J.d.P.; Linhares, A.C. Diversity of rotavirus strains circulating in Northern Brazil after introduction of a rotavirus vaccine: High prevalence of G3P[6] genotype. *J. Med. Virol.* **2014**, *86*, 1065–1072. [CrossRef]
13. Santos, V.S.; Nóbrega, F.A.; Soares, M.W.S.; Moreira, R.D.; Cuevas, L.E.; Gurgel, R.Q. Rotavirus genotypes circulating in Brazil before and after the national rotavirus vaccine program: A review. *Pediatr. Infect. Dis. J.* **2018**, *37*, e63–e65. [CrossRef]
14. Gutierrez, M.B.; Fialho, A.M.; Maranhão, A.G.; Malta, F.C.; Andrade, J.d.S.R.d.; de Assis, R.M.S.; Mouta, S.D.S.E.; Miagostovich, M.P.; Leite, J.P.G.; Machado Fumian, T. Rotavirus A in Brazil: Molecular epidemiology and surveillance during 2018–2019. *Pathogens* **2020**, *9*, 515. [CrossRef]
15. Gurgel, R.Q.; Cuevas, L.E.; Vieira, S.C.; Barros, V.C.; Fontes, P.B.; Salustino, E.F.; Nakagomi, O.; Nakagomi, T.; Dove, W.; Cunliffe, N.; et al. Predominance of rotavirus P[4]G2 in a vaccinated population, Brazil. *Emerg. Infect. Dis.* **2007**, *13*, 1571–1573. [CrossRef]
16. Nakagomi, T.; Cuevas, L.E.; Gurgel, R.G.; Elrokhsi, S.H.; Belkhir, Y.A.; Abugalia, M.; Dove, W.; Montenegro, F.M.U.; Correia, J.B.; Nakagomi, O.; et al. Apparent extinction of non-G2 rotavirus strains from circulation in Recife, Brazil, after the introduction of rotavirus vaccine. *Arch. Virol.* **2008**, *153*, 591–593. [CrossRef]
17. Montenegro, F.M.U.; Falbo, A.R.; Germano, E.M.; Correia, N.B.; Souza, E.d.S.; Nakagomi, O.; Nakagomi, T.; Cuevas, L.E.; Cunliffe, N.A.; Correia, J.B. Reduction in rotavirus disease and sustained predominance of G2P[4] rotavirus strain following introduction of rotavirus vaccine in Recife, Brazil. *J. Trop. Pediatr.* **2015**, *61*, 206–209. [CrossRef]

18. Kirkwood, C.D.; Boniface, K.; Bishop, R.F.; Barnes, G.L.; Australian Rotavirus Surveillance Group. Australian rotavirus surveillance program annual report, 2008/2009. *Commun. Dis. Intell. Q. Rep.* **2009**, *33*, 382–388. [CrossRef]
19. Patel, M.; Pedreira, C.; De Oliveira, L.H.; Tate, J.; Orozco, M.; Mercado, J.; Gonzalez, A.; Malespin, O.; Amador, J.J.; Umaña, J.; et al. Association between pentavalent rotavirus vaccine and severe rotavirus diarrhea among children in Nicaragua. *JAMA* **2009**, *301*, 2243–2251. [CrossRef] [PubMed]
20. Dóró, R.; László, B.; Martella, V.; Leshem, E.; Gentsch, J.; Parashar, U.; Bányai, K. Review of global rotavirus strain prevalence data from six years post vaccine licensure surveillance: Is there evidence of strain selection from vaccine pressure? *Infect. Genet. Evol.* **2014**, *28*, 446–461. [CrossRef] [PubMed]
21. Donato, C.M.; Zhang, Z.A.; Donker, N.C.; Kirkwood, C.D. Characterization of G2P[4] rotavirus strains associated with increased detection in Australian states using the RotaTeq® vaccine during the 2010–2011 surveillance period. *Infect. Genet. Evol.* **2014**, *28*, 398–412. [CrossRef] [PubMed]
22. Thanh, H.D.; Tran, V.T.; Lim, I.; Kim, W. Emergence of human G2P[4] rotaviruses in the post-vaccination era in South Korea: Footprints of multiple interspecies re-assortment events. *Sci. Rep.* **2018**, *8*, 6011. [CrossRef] [PubMed]
23. Antunes, H.; Afonso, A.; Iturriza, M.; Martinho, I.; Ribeiro, C.; Rocha, S.; Magalhães, C.; Carvalho, L.; Branca, F.; Gray, J. G2P[4] the most prevalent rotavirus genotype in 2007 winter season in an European non-vaccinated population. *J. Clin. Virol.* **2009**, *45*, 76–78. [CrossRef] [PubMed]
24. Martínez, M.; Amarilla, A.A.; Galeano, M.E.; Aquino, V.H.; Fariña, N.; Russomando, G.; Parra, G.I. Predominance of rotavirus G2P[4] and emergence of G12P[9] strains in Asunción, Paraguay, 2006–2007. *Arch. Virol.* **2010**, *155*, 525–533. [CrossRef]
25. Gurgel, R.Q.; Alvarez, A.D.J.; Rodrigues, A.; Ribeiro, R.R.; Dolabella, S.S.; Da Mota, N.L.; Santos, V.S.; Iturriza-Gomara, M.; Cunliffe, N.A.; Cuevas, L.E. Incidence of rotavirus and circulating genotypes in Northeast Brazil during 7 years of national rotavirus vaccination. *PLoS ONE* **2014**, *9*, e110217. [CrossRef]
26. Luchs, A.; Cilli, A.; Morillo, S.G.; de Cassia Compagnoli Carmona, R.; do Carmo Sampaio Tavares Timenetsky, M. Rotavirus in adults, Brazil, 2004–2011: G2P[4] dominance and potential impact on vaccination. *Braz. J. Infect. Dis.* **2014**, *18*, 53–59. [CrossRef]
27. Kirkwood, C.D.; Roczo-Farkas, S.; Bishop, R.F.; Barnes, G.L.; Australian Rotavirus Surveillance Group. Australian Rotavirus Surveillance Program annual report, 2013. *Commun. Dis. Intell. Q. Rep.* **2014**, *38*, E334–E342. [CrossRef]
28. Linhares, A.C.; Stupka, J.A.; Ciapponi, A.; Bardach, A.E.; Glujovsky, D.; Aruj, P.K.; Mazzoni, A.; Rodriguez, J.A.B.; Rearte, A.; Lanzieri, T.M.; et al. Burden and typing of rotavirus group A in Latin America and the Caribbean: Systematic review and meta-analysis. *Rev. Med. Virol.* **2011**, *21*, 89–109. [CrossRef]
29. Adah, M.I.; Wade, A.; Taniguchi, K. Molecular epidemiology of rotaviruses in Nigeria: Detection of unusual strains with G2P[6] and G8P[1] specificities. *J. Clin. Microbiol.* **2001**, *39*, 3969–3975. [CrossRef]
30. Clark, H.F.; Lawley, D.; DiStefano, D.; Maliga, M.; Kilby, B.; Kulnis, G.; Mallette, L.; DiNubile, M.J. An unusual outbreak of rotavirus genotype G2P[6] during the 2005–2006 epidemic season in Philadelphia. *Diagn. Microbiol. Infect. Dis.* **2011**, *70*, 218–222. [CrossRef]
31. Enweronu-Laryea, C.C.; Sagoe, K.W.; Damanka, S.; Lartey, B.; Armah, G.E. Rotavirus genotypes associated with childhood severe acute diarrhoea in southern Ghana: A cross-sectional study. *Virol. J.* **2013**, *10*, 287. [CrossRef]
32. Ghosh, S.; Urushibara, N.; Chawla-Sarkar, M.; Krishnan, T.; Kobayashi, N. Whole genomic analyses of asymptomatic human G1P[6], G2P[6] and G3P[6] rotavirus strains reveal intergenogroup reassortment events and genome segments of artiodactyl origin. *Infect. Genet. Evol.* **2013**, *16*, 165–173. [CrossRef]
33. Heylen, E.; Zeller, M.; Ciarlet, M.; De Coster, S.; Van Ranst, M.; Matthijnssens, J. Complete genetic characterization of human G2P[6] and G3P[6] rotavirus strains. *Infect. Genet. Evol.* **2013**, *13*, 27–35. [CrossRef] [PubMed]
34. Luchs, A.; Cilli, A.; Morillo, S.G.; Gregório, D.d.S.; de Souza, K.A.F.; Vieira, H.R.; Fernandes, A.d.M.; Carmona, R.d.C.C.; Timenetsky, M.d.C.S.T. Detection of the emerging rotavirus G12P[8] genotype at high frequency in Brazil in 2014: Successive replacement of predominant strains after vaccine introduction. *Acta Trop.* **2016**, *156*, 87–94. [CrossRef] [PubMed]
35. Agbla, J.M.; Esona, M.D.; Jaimes, J.; Gautam, R.; Agbankpé, A.J.; Katz, E.; Dougnon, T.V.; Capo-Chichi, A.; Ouedraogo, N.; Razack, O.; et al. Whole genome analysis of rotavirus strains circulating in Benin before vaccine introduction, 2016–2018. *Virus Res.* **2022**, *313*, 198715. [CrossRef] [PubMed]
36. Mwangi, P.N.; Potgieter, R.-L.; Simwaka, J.; Mpabalwani, E.M.; Mwenda, J.M.; Mogotsi, M.T.; Magagula, N.; Esona, M.D.; Steele, A.D.; Seheri, M.L.; et al. Genomic analysis of G2P[4] group A rotaviruses in Zambia reveals positive selection in amino acid site 7 of viral protein 3. *Viruses* **2023**, *15*, 501. [CrossRef]
37. Lestari, F.B.; Vongpunsawad, S.; Wanlapakorn, N.; Poovorawan, Y. Rotavirus infection in children in Southeast Asia 2008–2018: Disease burden, genotype distribution, seasonality, and vaccination. *J. Biomed. Sci.* **2020**, *27*, 66. [CrossRef]
38. Bányai, K.; Martella, V.; Jakab, F.; Melegh, B.; Szücs, G. Sequencing and phylogenetic analysis of human genotype P[6] rotavirus strains detected in Hungary provides evidence for genetic heterogeneity within the P[6] VP4 gene. *J. Clin. Microbiol.* **2004**, *42*, 4338–4343. [CrossRef] [PubMed]

39. Martella, V.; Bányai, K.; Ciarlet, M.; Iturriza-Gómara, M.; Lorusso, E.; De Grazia, S.; Arista, S.; Decaro, N.; Elia, G.; Cavalli, A.; et al. Relationships among porcine and human P[6] rotaviruses: Evidence that the different human P[6] lineages have originated from multiple interspecies transmission events. *Virology* **2006**, *344*, 509–519. [CrossRef]
40. Nyaga, M.M.; Tan, Y.; Seheri, M.L.; Halpin, R.A.; Akopov, A.; Stucker, K.M.; Fedorova, N.B.; Shrivastava, S.; Duncan Steele, A.; Mwenda, J.M.; et al. Whole-genome sequencing and analyses identify high genetic heterogeneity, diversity and endemicity of rotavirus genotype P[6] strains circulating in Africa. *Infect. Genet. Evol.* **2018**, *63*, 79–88. [CrossRef]
41. Linhares, A.C.; Mascarenhas, J.D.P.; Gusmão, R.H.P.; Gabbay, Y.B.; Fialho, A.M.; Leite, J.P.G. Neonatal rotavirus infection in Belém, northern Brazil: Nosocomial transmission of a P[6] G2 strain. *J. Med. Virol.* **2002**, *67*, 418–426. [CrossRef] [PubMed]
42. Mascarenhas, J.D.P.; Linhares, A.C.; Bayma, A.P.G.; Lima, J.C.; Sousa, M.S.; Araújo, I.T.; Heinemann, M.B.; Gusmão, R.H.P.; Gabbay, Y.B.; Leite, J.P.G. Molecular analysis of VP4, VP7, and NSP4 genes of P[6]G2 rotavirus genotype strains recovered from neonates admitted to hospital in Belém, Brazil. *J. Med. Virol.* **2006**, *78*, 281–289. [CrossRef] [PubMed]
43. Papp, H.; Borzák, R.; Farkas, S.; Kisfali, P.; Lengyel, G.; Molnár, P.; Melegh, B.; Matthijnssens, J.; Jakab, F.; Martella, V.; et al. Zoonotic transmission of reassortant porcine G4P[6] rotaviruses in Hungarian pediatric patients identified sporadically over a 15 year period. *Infect. Genet. Evol.* **2013**, *19*, 71–80. [CrossRef]
44. Luchs, A.; Timenetsky, M.D.C.S.T. G8P[6] rotaviruses isolated from Amerindian children in Mato Grosso do Sul, Brazil, during 2009: Close relationship of the G and P genes with those of bovine and bat strains. *J. Gen. Virol.* **2014**, *95*, 627–641. [CrossRef] [PubMed]
45. Lee, S.-K.; Oh, S.J.; Choi, S.; Choi, S.H.; Shin, S.-H.; Lee, E.J.; Cho, E.-J.; Hyun, J.; Kim, H.S. Relationship Between Rotavirus P[6] Infection in Korean Neonates and Histo-Blood Group Antigen: A Single-Center Study. *Ann. Lab. Med.* **2021**, *41*, 181–189. [CrossRef]
46. Herring, A.J.; Inglis, N.F.; Ojeh, C.K.; Snodgrass, D.R.; Menzies, J.D. Rapid diagnosis of rotavirus infection by direct detection of viral nucleic acid in silver-stained polyacrylamide gels. *J. Clin. Microbiol.* **1982**, *16*, 473–477. [CrossRef]
47. Mijatovic-Rustempasic, S.; Bányai, K.; Esona, M.D.; Foytich, K.; Bowen, M.D.; Gentsch, J.R. Genome sequence based molecular epidemiology of unusual US Rotavirus A G9 strains isolated from Omaha, USA between 1997 and 2000. *Infect. Genet. Evol.* **2011**, *11*, 522–527. [CrossRef]
48. Wang, Y.-H.; Pang, B.-B.; Ghosh, S.; Zhou, X.; Shintani, T.; Urushibara, N.; Song, Y.-W.; He, M.-Y.; Liu, M.-Q.; Tang, W.-F.; et al. Molecular epidemiology and genetic evolution of the whole genome of G3P[8] human rotavirus in Wuhan, China, from 2000 through 2013. *PLoS ONE* **2014**, *9*, e88850. [CrossRef]
49. Magagula, N.B.; Esona, M.D.; Nyaga, M.M.; Stucker, K.M.; Halpin, R.A.; Stockwell, T.B.; Seheri, M.L.; Steele, A.D.; Wentworth, D.E.; Mphahlele, M.J. Whole genome analyses of G1P[8] rotavirus strains from vaccinated and non-vaccinated South African children presenting with diarrhea. *J. Med. Virol.* **2015**, *87*, 79–101. [CrossRef]
50. Varghese, V.; Ghosh, S.; Das, S.; Bhattacharya, S.K.; Krishnan, T.; Karmakar, P.; Kobayashi, N.; Naik, T.N. Characterization of VP1, VP2 and VP3 gene segments of a human rotavirus closely related to porcine strains. *Virus Genes* **2006**, *32*, 241–247. [CrossRef]
51. Gentsch, J.R.; Glass, R.I.; Woods, P.; Gouvea, V.; Gorziglia, M.; Flores, J.; Das, B.K.; Bhan, M.K. Identification of group A rotavirus gene 4 types by polymerase chain reaction. *J. Clin. Microbiol.* **1992**, *30*, 1365–1373. [CrossRef]
52. Gouvea, V.; Glass, R.I.; Woods, P.; Taniguchi, K.; Clark, H.F.; Forrester, B.; Fang, Z.Y. Polymerase chain reaction amplification and typing of rotavirus nucleic acid from stool specimens. *J. Clin. Microbiol.* **1990**, *28*, 276–282. [CrossRef]
53. Kumar, S.; Stecher, G.; Li, M.; Knyaz, C.; Tamura, K. MEGA X: Molecular Evolutionary Genetics Analysis across Computing Platforms. *Mol. Biol. Evol.* **2018**, *35*, 1547–1549. [CrossRef]
54. Agbemabiese, C.A.; Nakagomi, T.; Damanka, S.A.; Dennis, F.E.; Lartey, B.L.; Armah, G.E.; Nakagomi, O. Sub-genotype phylogeny of the non-G, non-P genes of genotype 2 Rotavirus A strains. *PLoS ONE* **2019**, *14*, e0217422. [CrossRef]
55. Azevedo, L.S.; Costa, F.F.; Ghani, M.B.A.; Viana, E.; França, Y.; Medeiros, R.S.; Guiducci, R.; Morillo, S.G.; Primo, D.; Lopes, R.D.; et al. Full genotype characterization of Brazilian canine G3P[3] strains during a 10-year survey (2012–2021) of rotavirus infection in domestic dogs and cats. *Arch. Virol.* **2023**, *168*, 176. [CrossRef]
56. Gupta, S.; Gauhar, M.; Bubber, P.; Ray, P. Phylogenetic analysis of VP7 and VP4 genes of the most predominant human group A rotavirus G12 identified in children with acute gastroenteritis in Himachal Pradesh, India during 2013–2016. *J. Med. Virol.* **2021**, *93*, 6200–6209. [CrossRef]
57. Doan, Y.H.; Nakagomi, T.; Agbemabiese, C.A.; Nakagomi, O. Changes in the distribution of lineage constellations of G2P[4] Rotavirus A strains detected in Japan over 32 years (1980–2011). *Infect. Genet. Evol.* **2015**, *34*, 423–433. [CrossRef] [PubMed]
58. Heylen, E.; Zeller, M.; Ciarlet, M.; Lawrence, J.; Steele, D.; Van Ranst, M.; Matthijnssens, J. Comparative analysis of pentavalent rotavirus vaccine strains and G8 rotaviruses identified during vaccine trial in Africa. *Sci. Rep.* **2015**, *5*, 14658. [CrossRef]
59. Jere, K.C.; Chaguza, C.; Bar-Zeev, N.; Lowe, J.; Peno, C.; Kumwenda, B.; Nakagomi, O.; Tate, J.E.; Parashar, U.D.; Heyderman, R.S.; et al. Emergence of Double- and Triple-Gene Reassortant G1P[8] Rotaviruses Possessing a DS-1-Like Backbone after Rotavirus Vaccine Introduction in Malawi. *J. Virol.* **2018**, *92*, e01246-17. [CrossRef] [PubMed]
60. Munlela, B.; João, E.D.; Strydom, A.; Bauhofer, A.F.L.; Chissaque, A.; Chilaúle, J.J.; Maurício, I.L.; Donato, C.M.; O'Neill, H.G.; de Deus, N. Whole-Genome Characterization of Rotavirus G9P[6] and G9P[4] Strains That Emerged after Rotavirus Vaccine Introduction in Mozambique. *Viruses* **2024**, *16*, 1140. [CrossRef] [PubMed]

61. Rahman, M.; Matthijnssens, J.; Yang, X.; Delbeke, T.; Arijs, I.; Taniguchi, K.; Iturriza-Gómara, M.; Iftekharuddin, N.; Azim, T.; Van Ranst, M. Evolutionary history and global spread of the emerging g12 human rotaviruses. *J. Virol.* **2007**, *81*, 2382–2390. [CrossRef]
62. Sharma, S.; Paul, V.K.; Bhan, M.K.; Ray, P. Genomic characterization of nontypeable rotaviruses and detection of a rare G8 strain in Delhi, India. *J. Clin. Microbiol.* **2009**, *47*, 3998–4005. [CrossRef]
63. De Grazia, S.; Giammanco, G.M.; Dóró, R.; Bonura, F.; Marton, S.; Cascio, A.; Martella, V.; Bányai, K. Identification of a multi-reassortant G12P[9] rotavirus with novel VP1, VP2, VP3 and NSP2 genotypes in a child with acute gastroenteritis. *Infect. Genet. Evol.* **2015**, *35*, 34–37. [CrossRef]
64. Doan, Y.H.; Dennis, F.E.; Takemae, N.; Haga, K.; Shimizu, H.; Appiah, M.G.; Lartey, B.L.; Damanka, S.A.; Hayashi, T.; Suzuki, T.; et al. Emergence of Intergenogroup Reassortant G9P[4] Strains Following Rotavirus Vaccine Introduction in Ghana. *Viruses* **2023**, *15*, 2453. [CrossRef] [PubMed]
65. Lewis, J.; Roy, S.; Esona, M.D.; Mijatovic-Rustempasic, S.; Hardy, C.; Wang, Y.; Cortese, M.; Bowen, M.D. Full Genome Sequence of a Reassortant Human G9P[4] Rotavirus Strain. *Genome Announc.* **2014**, *2*, e01284-14. [CrossRef] [PubMed]
66. Doan, Y.H.; Suzuki, Y.; Fujii, Y.; Haga, K.; Fujimoto, A.; Takai-Todaka, R.; Someya, Y.; Nayak, M.K.; Mukherjee, A.; Imamura, D.; et al. Complex reassortment events of unusual G9P[4] rotavirus strains in India between 2011 and 2013. *Infect. Genet. Evol.* **2017**, *54*, 417–428. [CrossRef]
67. Quaye, O.; McDonald, S.; Esona, M.D.; Lyde, F.C.; Mijatovic-Rustempasic, S.; Roy, S.; Banegas, D.J.C.; Quiñonez, Y.M.; Chinchilla, B.L.; Santiago, F.G.; et al. Rotavirus G9P[4] in 3 countries in Latin America, 2009–2010. *Emerg. Infect. Dis.* **2013**, *19*, 1332–1333. [CrossRef]
68. Gutierrez, M.B.; de Assis, R.M.S.; Andrade, J.d.S.R.d.; Fialho, A.M.; Fumian, T.M. Rotavirus A during the COVID-19 Pandemic in Brazil, 2020–2022: Emergence of G6P[8] Genotype. *Viruses* **2023**, *15*, 1619. [CrossRef]
69. Medeiros, R.S.; França, Y.; Viana, E.; de Azevedo, L.S.; Guiducci, R.; de Lima Neto, D.F.; da Costa, A.C.; Luchs, A. Genomic Constellation of Human Rotavirus G8 Strains in Brazil over a 13-Year Period: Detection of the Novel Bovine-like G8P[8] Strains with the DS-1-like Backbone. *Viruses* **2023**, *15*, 664. [CrossRef]
70. França, Y.; Medeiros, R.S.; Viana, E.; de Azevedo, L.S.; Guiducci, R.; da Costa, A.C.; Luchs, A. Genetic diversity and evolution of G12P[6] DS-1-like and G12P[9] AU-1-like Rotavirus strains in Brazil. *Funct. Integr. Genom.* **2024**, *24*, 92. [CrossRef] [PubMed]
71. Moutelíková, R.; Sauer, P.; Prodělalová, J. Whole-genome sequence of a reassortant G9P[4] rotavirus A strain from two children in the Czech Republic. *Arch. Virol.* **2020**, *165*, 1703–1706. [CrossRef] [PubMed]
72. Kachooei, A.; Tava Koli, A.; Minaeian, S.; Hosseini, M.; Jalilvand, S.; Latifi, T.; Arashkia, A.; Ataei-Pirkooh, A.; Shoja, Z. Molecular characterization of rotavirus infections in children less than 5 years of age with acute gastroenteritis in Tehran, Iran, 2021–2022: Emergence of uncommon G9P[4] and G9P[8] rotavirus strains. *J. Med. Virol.* **2023**, *95*, e28529. [CrossRef]
73. Doan, Y.H.; Nakagomi, T.; Cunliffe, N.A.; Pandey, B.D.; Sherchand, J.B.; Nakagomi, O. The occurrence of amino acid substitutions D96N and S242N in VP7 of emergent G2P[4] rotaviruses in Nepal in 2004–2005: A global and evolutionary perspective. *Arch. Virol.* **2011**, *156*, 1969–1978. [CrossRef]
74. Dennis, A.F.; McDonald, S.M.; Payne, D.C.; Mijatovic-Rustempasic, S.; Esona, M.D.; Edwards, K.M.; Chappell, J.D.; Patton, J.T. Molecular epidemiology of contemporary G2P[4] human rotaviruses cocirculating in a single U.S. community: Footprints of a globally transitioning genotype. *J. Virol.* **2014**, *88*, 3789–3801. [CrossRef]
75. Pietsch, C.; Schuster, V.; Liebert, U.G. A hospital based study on inter- and intragenotypic diversity of human rotavirus A VP4 and VP7 gene segments, Germany. *J. Clin. Virol.* **2011**, *50*, 136–141. [CrossRef]
76. Do, L.P.; Nakagomi, T.; Doan, Y.H.; Kitahori, Y.; Nakagomi, O. Molecular evolution of the VP7 gene of Japanese G2 rotaviruses before vaccine introduction. *Arch. Virol.* **2014**, *159*, 315–319. [CrossRef]
77. Wu, F.-T.; Bányai, K.; Jiang, B.; Wu, C.-Y.; Chen, H.-C.; Fehér, E.; Huang, Y.-C.; Lin, J.-S.; Huang, F.-C.; Hsiung, C.A.; et al. Molecular epidemiology of human G2P[4] rotaviruses in Taiwan, 2004–2011. *Infect. Genet. Evol.* **2014**, *28*, 530–536. [CrossRef]
78. Paul, S.K.; Kobayashi, N.; Nagashima, S.; Ishino, M.; Watanabe, S.; Alam, M.M.; Ahmed, M.U.; Hossain, M.A.; Naik, T.N. Phylogenetic analysis of rotaviruses with genotypes G1, G2, G9 and G12 in Bangladesh: Evidence for a close relationship between rotaviruses from children and adults. *Arch. Virol.* **2008**, *153*, 1999–2012. [CrossRef]
79. Nakagomi, T.; Doan, Y.H.; Dove, W.; Ngwira, B.; Iturriza-Gómara, M.; Nakagomi, O.; Cunliffe, N.A. G8 rotaviruses with conserved genotype constellations detected in Malawi over 10 years (1997–2007) display frequent gene reassortment among strains co-circulating in humans. *J. Gen. Virol.* **2013**, *94*, 1273–1295. [CrossRef] [PubMed]
80. Ndze, V.N.; Esona, M.D.; Achidi, E.A.; Gonsu, K.H.; Dóró, R.; Marton, S.; Farkas, S.; Ngeng, M.B.; Ngu, A.F.; Obama-Abena, M.T.; et al. Full genome characterization of human Rotavirus A strains isolated in Cameroon, 2010–2011: Diverse combinations of the G and P genes and lack of reassortment of the backbone genes. *Infect. Genet. Evol.* **2014**, *28*, 537–560. [CrossRef] [PubMed]
81. Langa, J.S.; Thompson, R.; Arnaldo, P.; Resque, H.R.; Rose, T.; Enosse, S.M.; Fialho, A.; de Assis, R.M.S.; da Silva, M.F.M.; Leite, J.P.G. Epidemiology of rotavirus A diarrhea in Chókwè, Southern Mozambique, from February to September, 2011. *J. Med. Virol.* **2016**, *88*, 1751–1758. [CrossRef] [PubMed]

82. Martinez, M.; Galeano, M.E.; Akopov, A.; Palacios, R.; Russomando, G.; Kirkness, E.F.; Parra, G.I. Whole-genome analyses reveals the animal origin of a rotavirus G4P[6] detected in a child with severe diarrhea. *Infect. Genet. Evol.* **2014**, *27*, 156–162. [CrossRef]
83. Malasao, R.; Khamrin, P.; Kumthip, K.; Ushijima, H.; Maneekarn, N. Complete genome sequence analysis of rare G4P[6] rotavirus strains from human and pig reveals the evidence for interspecies transmission. *Infect. Genet. Evol.* **2018**, *65*, 357–368. [CrossRef]
84. Gutierrez, M.B.; de Assis, R.M.S.; Arantes, I.; Fumian, T.M. Full genotype constellations analysis of unusual DS-1-like G12P[6] and G6P[8] rotavirus strains detected in Brazil, 2019. *Virology* **2022**, *577*, 74–83. [CrossRef]
85. Silva Serra, A.C.; Júnior, E.C.; Cruz, J.F.; Lobo, P.S.; Júnior, E.T.; Bandeira, R.S.; Bezerra, D.A.; Mascarenhas, J.D.; Santos Guerra, S.F.; Soares, L.S. Molecular analysis of G3P[6] rotavirus in the Amazon region of Brazil: Evidence of reassortment with equine-like strains. *Future Microbiol.* **2021**, *16*, 847–862. [CrossRef]
86. Giammanco, G.M.; Bonura, F.; Zeller, M.; Heylen, E.; Van Ranst, M.; Martella, V.; Bányai, K.; Matthijnssens, J.; De Grazia, S. Evolution of DS-1-like human G2P[4] rotaviruses assessed by complete genome analyses. *J. Gen. Virol.* **2014**, *95*, 91–109. [CrossRef]
87. Aida, S.; Nahar, S.; Paul, S.K.; Hossain, M.A.; Kabir, M.R.; Sarkar, S.R.; Ahmed, S.; Ghosh, S.; Urushibara, N.; Kawaguchiya, M.; et al. Whole genomic analysis of G2P[4] human Rotaviruses in Mymensingh, north-central Bangladesh. *Heliyon* **2016**, *2*, e00168. [CrossRef]
88. Gómez, M.M.; Carvalho-Costa, F.A.; Volotão, E.d.M.; Rose, T.L.; da Silva, M.F.M.; Fialho, A.M.; de Assis, R.M.S.; Andrade, J.d.S.R.d.; Sá, A.C.C.; Zeller, M.; et al. Prevalence and genomic characterization of G2P[4] group A rotavirus strains during monovalent vaccine introduction in Brazil. *Infect. Genet. Evol.* **2014**, *28*, 486–494. [CrossRef] [PubMed]
89. Silva-Sales, M.; Leal, E.; Milagres, F.A.d.P.; Brustulin, R.; Morais, V.D.S.; Marcatti, R.; Araújo, E.L.L.; Witkin, S.S.; Deng, X.; Sabino, E.C.; et al. Genomic constellation of human Rotavirus A strains identified in Northern Brazil: A 6-year follow-up (2010–2016). *Rev. Inst. Med. Trop. Sao Paulo* **2020**, *62*, e98. [CrossRef]
90. Dóró, R.; Mihalov-Kovács, E.; Marton, S.; László, B.; Deák, J.; Jakab, F.; Juhász, Á.; Kisfali, P.; Martella, V.; Melegh, B.; et al. Large-scale whole genome sequencing identifies country-wide spread of an emerging G9P[8] rotavirus strain in Hungary, 2012. *Infect. Genet. Evol.* **2014**, *28*, 495–512. [CrossRef] [PubMed]
91. Tacharoenmuang, R.; Komoto, S.; Guntapong, R.; Ide, T.; Sinchai, P.; Upachai, S.; Yoshikawa, T.; Tharmaphornpilas, P.; Sangkitporn, S.; Taniguchi, K. Full Genome Characterization of Novel DS-1-Like G8P[8] Rotavirus Strains that Have Emerged in Thailand: Reassortment of Bovine and Human Rotavirus Gene Segments in Emerging DS-1-Like Intergenogroup Reassortant Strains. *PLoS ONE* **2016**, *11*, e0165826. [CrossRef] [PubMed]
92. Morozova, O.V.; Sashina, T.A.; Epifanova, N.V.; Velikzhanina, E.I.; Novikova, N.A. Phylodynamic characteristics of reassortant DS-1-like G3P[8]-strains of rotavirus type A isolated in Nizhny Novgorod (Russia). *Braz. J. Microbiol.* **2023**, *54*, 2867–2877. [CrossRef] [PubMed]
93. Pradhan, G.N.; Walimbe, A.M.; Chitambar, S.D. Molecular characterization of emerging G9P[4] rotavirus strains possessing a rare E6 NSP4 or T1 NSP3 genotype on a genogroup-2 backbone using a refined classification framework. *J. Gen. Virol.* **2016**, *97*, 3139–3153. [CrossRef]
94. Komoto, S.; Tacharoenmuang, R.; Guntapong, R.; Ide, T.; Haga, K.; Katayama, K.; Kato, T.; Ouchi, Y.; Kurahashi, H.; Tsuji, T.; et al. Emergence and Characterization of Unusual DS-1-Like G1P[8] Rotavirus Strains in Children with Diarrhea in Thailand. *PLoS ONE* **2015**, *10*, e0141739. [CrossRef]
95. Pietsch, C.; Liebert, U.G. Molecular characterization of different equine-like G3 rotavirus strains from Germany. *Infect. Genet. Evol.* **2018**, *57*, 46–50. [CrossRef]
96. Luchs, A.; da Costa, A.C.; Cilli, A.; Komninakis, S.C.V.; Carmona, R.d.C.C.; Boen, L.; Morillo, S.G.; Sabino, E.C.; Timenetsky, M.D.C.S.T. Spread of the emerging equine-like G3P[8] DS-1-like genetic backbone rotavirus strain in Brazil and identification of potential genetic variants. *J. Gen. Virol.* **2019**, *100*, 7–25. [CrossRef]
97. Komoto, S.; Tacharoenmuang, R.; Guntapong, R.; Ide, T.; Tsuji, T.; Yoshikawa, T.; Tharmaphornpilas, P.; Sangkitporn, S.; Taniguchi, K. Reassortment of Human and Animal Rotavirus Gene Segments in Emerging DS-1-Like G1P[8] Rotavirus Strains. *PLoS ONE* **2016**, *11*, e0148416. [CrossRef]
98. Fujii, Y.; Doan, Y.H.; Suzuki, Y.; Nakagomi, T.; Nakagomi, O.; Katayama, K. Study of Complete Genome Sequences of Rotavirus A Epidemics and Evolution in Japan in 2012–2014. *Front. Microbiol.* **2019**, *10*, 38. [CrossRef]
99. Luchs, A.; da Costa, A.C.; Cilli, A.; Komninakis, S.C.V.; Carmona, R.d.C.C.; Morillo, S.G.; Sabino, E.C.; Timenetsky, M.d.C.S.T. First Detection of DS-1-like G1P[8] Double-gene Reassortant Rotavirus Strains on The American Continent, Brazil, 2013. *Sci. Rep.* **2019**, *9*, 2210. [CrossRef] [PubMed]

viruses

MDPI

Article

Epidemiological and Genetic Characteristics of Sapovirus in Shandong, China, 2022–2023

Mingxin Guo [1,2,†], Meijia Li [1,†], Ti Liu [2,3], Wenkui Sun [2,3], Kaige Du [2,3], Shuopeng Yang [2,3], Zhongyan Fu [2,3,*] and Zengqiang Kou [2,3,*]

1 School of Public Health and Health Management, Shandong First Medical University, Shandong Academy of Medical Sciences, Jinan 250117, China; gmx15610398290@163.com (M.G.); 15666250190@163.com (M.L.)

2 Shandong Provincial Center for Disease Control and Prevention, Jinan 250014, China; liuti1204@126.com (T.L.); wenkuisun@163.com (W.S.); 18369607969@163.com (K.D.); yyysp123456@163.com (S.Y.)

3 Shandong Provincial Key Laboratory of Intelligent Monitoring, Early Warning, Prevention and Control for Infectious Diseases, Jinan 250014, China

* Correspondence: zhongyanfu@163.com (Z.F.); jack-cou@163.com (Z.K.)

† These authors contributed equally to this work.

Abstract: Sapovirus (SaV) is a major pathogen responsible for acute gastroenteritis (AGE), and its incidence has been increasing in recent years. This study investigates the prevalence and the genetic characteristics of SaV in Shandong Province during 2022–2023, based on a surveillance network covering all age groups. Samples were obtained from a viral diarrhea surveillance network in Shandong Province during 2022–2023. SaVs were identified through quantitative reverse-transcription polymerase chain reaction (RT-qPCR). PCR amplification and Sanger sequencing were performed on positive samples, and whole-genome sequencing was conducted using metagenomic sequencing technology. Sequence analysis was conducted using BioEdit 7.0.9.0 and MEGA X, while statistical analysis was performed with SPSS 26.0. A total of 157 SaV-positive cases were identified, resulting in a positivity rate of 1.12%. The positivity rate for SaV was 0.75% in 2022 and it increased significantly to 1.42% in 2023. The highest positivity rates for both 2022 and 2023 were observed in November. The highest positivity rate was observed in the 3–5-year-old age group. In 2022, Dongying City had the highest positivity rate, while Zaozhuang City exhibited the highest rate in 2023. The incidence of vomiting in SaV-positive patients was significantly higher compared to SaV-negative patients ($P = 0.002$). Eight genotypes were identified in both the VP1 and RdRp regions. The complete genome sequence analysis of a GI.3 strain showed that NS1 (5.88%, 4/68) was the region most prone to amino acid variation, followed by VP2 (5.45%, 9/165) within the same genotype. SaV infections are more prevalent in cold weather, with young children being particularly susceptible. The SaV positivity rate in 2023 increased significantly accompanied by an increased diversity of genotypes, compared to that of 2022. The NS1 region exhibits the biggest variation within the same genotype, indicating that more attention should be paid to other regions besides VP1 in the future study. Ongoing surveillance of SaV is recommended for effective prevention and control.

Keywords: sapovirus; epidemiology; genotypes; genome analysis

1. Introduction

Sapovirus (SaV) was first identified in human fecal samples in 1976 using electron microscopy [1]. It is a significant pathogen responsible for acute gastroenteritis (AGE), characterized by clinical symptoms such as fever, nausea, vomiting, diarrhea, abdominal pain, and abdominal cramps [2]. SaV can infect individuals across all age groups, with children being the most commonly affected population [3–5]. SaV can cause both sporadic infections and outbreaks [6,7]. In recent years, following the end of the COVID-19 pandemic, an increase in SaV incidence was observed [8]. Furthermore, studies from countries that have incorporated the rotavirus vaccine into their immunization programs showed an increasing trend of SaV infection [9].

A member of the Caliciviridae family, SaV has a single-stranded, positive-sense RNA genome approximately 7.1–7.7 kb in length, containing 2–3 open reading frames (ORFs). Recent studies have established a dual-typing classification system for SaV based on the complete nucleotide sequences of the RdRp and VP1 regions [10]. This system identifies 34 genogroups and 24 P-genogroups. Among the genogroups that infect humans (GI, GII, GIV, and GV), 20 genotypes (GI.1-7, GII.1-8, GII.NA1, GIV.1, GV.1-2, and GV.NA1) and 21 P-genotypes (GI.P1-P3, GI.P5-P7, GII.P1-P10, GII.PNA1-PNA2, GV.P1-P2, and GV.PNA1) have been identified.

In Shandong Province, a viral diarrhea surveillance network covering all age groups was founded in 2016 and SaV was included in the surveillance in 2022. Each county investigated 3–5 cases of viral diarrhea per month and collected fecal samples to obtain pathological data. This study analyzed infections and the genetic characteristics of SaV in Shandong Province during 2022–2023. The epidemiological and pathogenic characteristics of SaV were identified.

2. Materials and Methods

2.1. Sample Source

A viral diarrhea surveillance network was implemented in 136 counties spanning all 16 cities of Shandong Province. Each county was monitored for three to five cases of viral diarrhea per month. Demographic data were collected through epidemiological surveys, and key clinical symptoms—including fever, nausea, vomiting, diarrhea, and abdominal pain—were systematically documented. Furthermore, fecal samples were systematically collected. Over the surveillance period from 1 January 2022 to 31 December 2023, a total of 14,011 case records and corresponding stool specimens were collected, of which 157 cases tested positive for SaV infection.

2.2. RNA Extraction and SaV RT-qPCR Detection

Fecal samples were processed to a 10% stool suspension using a Phosphate-Buffered Saline (PBS) buffer. Nucleic acid extraction was performed by 136 county-level Centers for Disease Control and Prevention (CDCs)in Shandong Province using several different nucleic acid extraction kits, followed by SaV detection. The extracted nucleic acids were subsequently transferred to municipal CDCs for SaV detection to ensure the accuracy of the results. SaV detection was performed using a commercial RT-qPCR kit (MABSKY, Shenzhen, China). The nucleic acid and test results were ultimately sent to the provincial CDC for compilation and analysis.

2.3. Genotype Identification

The RdRp and VP1 regions of SaV-positive samples were subsequently amplified according to Oka et al. [3]. The RdRp region of SaV-positive samples was amplified by RT-PCR using the SuperScript™ III One-Step RT-PCR with Platinum™ Taq kit (Invitrogen, Thermo Fisher Scientific, Waltham, MA, USA). The PCR amplification mixture contained 5 μL of template RNA, 15 μL of 2× reaction mix, 0.9 μL of each forward primer p290h (5′-GATTACTCCAGGTGGGACTCCAC-3′), p290i (5′-

GATTACTCCAGGTGGGACTCAAC-3′) and p290j (5′-GATTACTCCAGGTGGGATTCAAC-3′), p290k (5′-GATTACTCCAGGTGGGATTCCAC-3′), 1.2 μL of each reverse primer p289h (5′-TGACGATTTCATCATCACCATA-3′) and p289i (5′-TGACGATTTCATCATCCCCGTA-3′), 1.2 μL of Taq mix, and 2.8 μL of RNase-free water. The amplification conditions were 50 °C for 30 min reverse transcription, initial denaturation at 94 °C for 2 min, then 38 cycles of 94 °C for 30 s denaturation, 55 °C for 30 s for primer annealing, 68 °C for 1 min for extension, and finally 68 °C for 7 min for late extension. The expected PCR product size was 331 bp. The VP1 region of SaV-positive samples was amplified through an RT-nested PCR protocol. The first round of amplification was performed using the same kit as for the RdRp region. The PCR reaction mixture contained 5 μL of template RNA, 10 μL of 2× reaction mix, 0.6 μL of each forward primer SaV124F (5′-GAYCASGCTCTCGCYACCTAC-3′) and SaV1F (5′-TTGGCCCTCGCCACCTAC-3′), SaV5F (5′-TTTGAACAAGCTGTGGCATGCTAC-3′) and each reverse primer SV-R13 (5′-GGTGANAYNCCATTKTCCAT-3′) and SV-R14 (5′-GGTGAGMMYCCATTCTCCAT-3′), 0.8 μL of Taq mix, and 1.2 μL of RNase-free water. The thermal cycling conditions were as follows: initial denaturation at 94 °C for 3 min, followed by 35 cycles of denaturation at 94 °C for 30 s, annealing at 50 °C for 30 s, and extension at 72 °C for 1 min, with a final extension at 72 °C for 7 min. The second round of amplification was performed using the Platinum™ Taq DNA Polymerase kit (Invitrogen). The PCR reaction mixture contained 2 μL of 10× PCR Buffer-Mg, 0.6 μL of 50Mm $MgCl_2$, 0.4 μL of 10Mm dNTP mix, 0.4 μL of forward primer 1245Rfwd (5′-TAGTGTTTGARATGGAGGG-3′), reverse primer SV-R2 (5′- GWGGGRTCAACMCCWGGTGG-3′), 0.08 μL of Taq DNA Polymerase, 1 μL of the first-round PCR product, and 15.12 μL of RNase-free water. The thermal cycling conditions were as follows: reverse transcription at 50 °C for 30 min, initial denaturation at 94 °C for 2 min, followed by 40 cycles of denaturation at 94 °C for 30 s, annealing at 55 °C for 30 s, and extension at 68 °C for 1 min, with a final extension at 68 °C for 7 min. The expected PCR product size was 440 bp. The PCR products were sent to Sangon Biotechnology (Shanghai) Co., Ltd. for Sanger sequencing. The nucleotide sequences were used for genotype identification through phylogenetic analysis with reference sequences by Zhao et al. [10].

2.4. Next-Generation Sequencing (NGS)

Complete-genome sequencing of SaV was conducted using metagenomic sequencing technology. Library preparation was carried out with the VAHTS Universal V8 RNA-seq Library Prep Kit for Illumina (Vazyme, Nanjing, China) following the manufacturer's protocol. The prepared library was sequenced on an Illumina NextSeq 2000 platform (Illumina, San Diego, CA, USA) for high-throughput analysis. Raw sequencing data were assembled using the self-built workflow in CLC Genomics Workbench V21.0.2 (https://www.qiagenbioinformatics.com) (accessed on 18 October 2024), and the finalized sequences were deposited in the GenBank database (PV014972).

2.5. Sequence Analysis

The nucleotide and amino acid sequences were aligned using the ClustalW Multiple Alignment tool in BioEdit 7.0.9.0 [11]. Phylogenetic trees were constructed to illustrate genetic relationships using the Maximum Likelihood (ML) method with the Kimura 2-parameter nucleotide substitution model in MEGA X [12]. The reliability of the phylogenetic analysis was assessed with bootstrap values based on 1000 replicates.

2.6. Statistical Analysis

Epidemiological data were compiled using Excel 2021 (https://www.microsoft.com) (accessed on 1 January 2023), while statistical analyses were conducted with SPSS 26.0 (https://www.ibm.com/products/spss-statistics) (accessed on 1 January 2023). Categorical data were presented as rates or proportions. Group comparisons were performed using the chi-square test, with a significance level set at $\alpha = 0.05$. $P < 0.05$ was considered statistically significant.

3. Results

This study analyzed 14,011 cases and identified 157 SaV-positive cases, resulting in a positivity rate of 1.12%.

3.1. Temporal, Age, and Spatial Distribution

The positivity rate for SaV was 0.75% (47/6,290) in 2022 and it increased significantly to 1.42% (110/7,721) in 2023 ($\chi^2 = 14.358$, $P < 0.05$). Except for April 2022, SaV was identified in all other months. The highest positivity rates occurred in November of both years, reaching 1.50% in 2022 and 2.63% in 2023, as detailed in Table 1 and Figure 1.

Table 1. Monthly distribution of SaV infection cases.

Month	2022			2023		
	Cases (N)	Positive Cases (N)	SaV Positivity Rate (%)	Cases (N)	Positive Cases (N)	SaV Positivity Rate (%)
1	417	2	0.48	471	2	0.42
2	538	5	0.93	632	4	0.63
3	489	1	0.20	638	5	0.78
4	465	0	0	649	10	1.54
5	581	2	0.34	714	10	1.40
6	701	7	1.00	763	11	1.44
7	655	9	1.37	741	12	1.62
8	582	4	0.69	734	12	1.63
9	530	5	0.94	659	8	1.21
10	499	3	0.60	674	11	1.63
11	466	7	1.50	570	15	2.63
12	367	2	0.54	476	10	2.10
Total	6290	47	0.75	7721	110	1.42

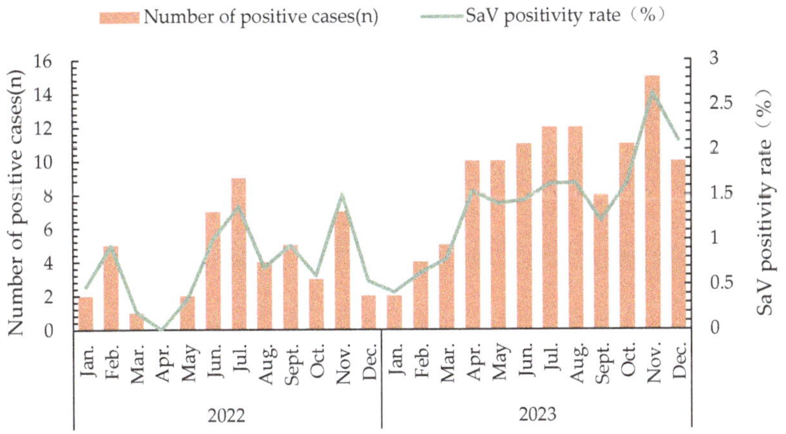

Figure 1. Temporal distribution of SaV infections in 2022–2023.

SaV was detected across all age groups. The highest positivity rate, 2.37%, was observed in the 3–5-year-old age group, primarily comprising preschool children, followed by 1.89% in the 12–17-year-old age group. The differences in SaV positivity rates among age groups were statistically significant ($\chi^2 = 47.289$, $P < 0.05$), as detailed in Table 2.

Table 2. Detection of SaV in different age groups.

Age (Years)	Cases (N)	Positive Cases (N)	SaV Positivity Rate (%)	χ^2	*P*-Value
0–2	3809	56	1.47	47.289	<0.05
3–5	1394	33	2.37		
6–11	923	13	1.41		
12–17	689	13	1.89		
18–59	4461	29	0.65		
≥60	2735	13	0.48		
Total	14,011	157	1.12		

The detection of SaV across cities in Shandong Province from 2022 to 2023 is shown in Figure 2. In 2022, Dongying City exhibited the highest positivity rate, at 2.30%. In 2023, Zaozhuang City recorded the highest positivity rate, reaching 5.38%.

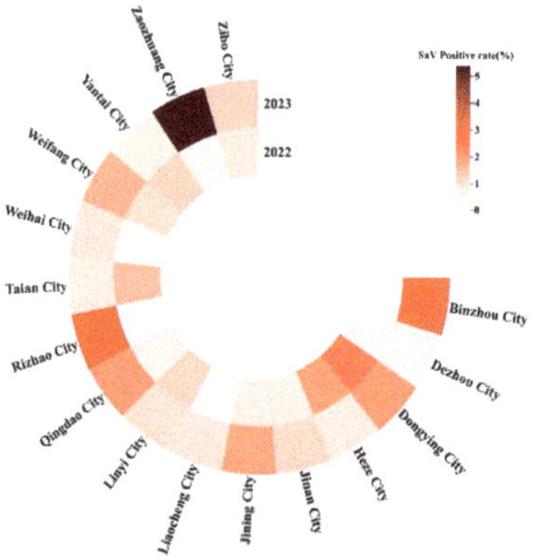

Figure 2. Detection of SaV across 16 cities in Shandong, 2022–2023. The color gradient in the legend, ranging from light to dark, represents an increasing SaV positivity rate, with lighter shades indicating lower rates and darker shades denoting higher rates.

3.2. *Clinical Manifestation*

Among the 14,011 cases, 195 records were excluded due to incompleteness or invalidity, leaving 13,816 cases for analysis. Of these, 11,458 (83%) were outpatient cases, and 2358 (17%) were inpatient cases. The SaV positivity rate was 1.09% for outpatients and 1.27% for inpatients. A comparison of SaV positivity rates between outpatient and inpatient cases revealed no statistically significant difference (χ^2 = 0.580, P = 0.446), as shown in Table 3.

Table 3. Comparison of SaV detection rates between outpatients and inpatients.

Type of Medical Visit	Cases (N)	Positive Cases (N)	SaV Positivity Rate (%)	χ^2	*P*-Value
Outpatients	11,458	125	1.09	0.580	0.446
Inpatients	2358	30	1.27		
Total	13,816	155	1.12		

As for symptoms, the incidence of vomiting is significantly higher in SaV-positive patients, compared to SaV-negative patients (P = 0.002). However, no statistically significant differences were observed in the incidence of other symptoms between the two groups (Table 4).

Table 4. Comparison of clinical symptoms between SaV-positive and SaV-negative patients.

Clinical Symptoms	SaV-Positive	SaV-Negative	χ^2	*P*-Value
Fever				
Yes	41	2892	2.575	0.109
No	116	10,962		
Nausea				
Yes	32	2890	0.022	0.883
No	125	10,964		
Vomiting				
Yes	53	3227	9.482	0.002
No	104	10,627		
Diarrhea				
Yes	147	13,240	1.369	0.242
No	10	614		
Abdominal pain				
Yes	53	5377	1.671	0.196
No	104	8477		

3.3. Genotype Distribution

Sequencing of the VP1 region was successfully performed on 90 samples, revealing eight genotypes: GI.1 (28 strains), GI.2 (15 strains), GI.3 (2 strains), GI.6 (8 strains), GII.1 (10 strains), GII.3 (10 strains), GII.5 (14 strains), and GIV.1 (3 strains). Sequencing of the RdRp region was successful for 68 samples, identifying eight P-genotypes: GI.P1 (25 strains), GI.P2 (10 strains), GI.P3 (2 strains), GI.P6 (5 strains), GII.P1 (10 strains), GII.P3 (10 strains), GII.P5 (4 strains), and GII.P10 (2 strains). The phylogenetic analyses are shown in Figure 3. Combined genotyping of the VP1 and RdRp regions identified 66 strains that were successfully detected in both regions, of which GI.1[P1] was the most common (37.88%, 25/66).

In 2022, five genotypes and five P-genotypes were identified, with GI.1 and GI.2 being the most frequently detected in VP1 region and GI.P1 being the most common in RdRp region. In 2023, eight genotypes and eight P-genotypes were detected. The most frequently identified genotypes were GI.1 and P-genotypes were GI.P1. The details are presented in Appendix A Table A1.

A

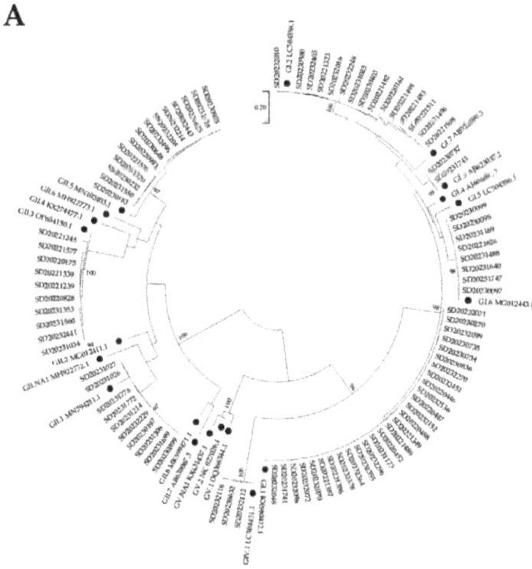

Figure 3. *Cont.*

B

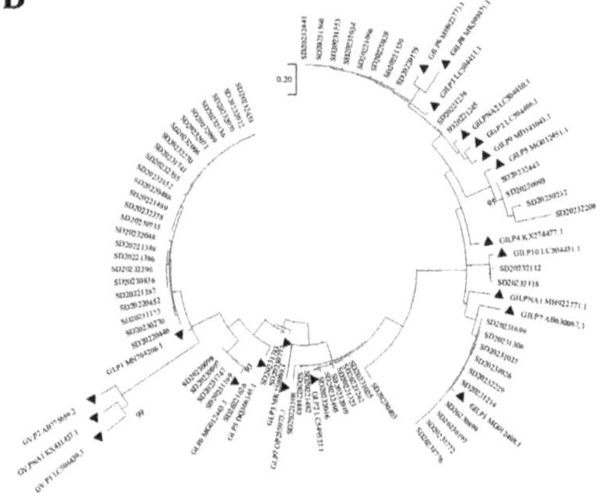

Figure 3. Phylogenetic analysis of nucleotide sequences in the SaV VP1 and RdRp regions. (**A**) • indicates the reference sequences of VP1 region. The sequence length was 274 bp of the partial VP1 region. (**B**) ▲ indicates the reference sequences of RdRp region. The sequence length was 132 bp of the partial RdRp region.

3.4. Analysis of Amino Acid Variation Characteristics

Given the scarcity of complete GI.3 SaV genomes in GenBank (only eleven available), metagenomic sequencing was performed on two GI.3 SaV strains obtained in this study, with only one successfully sequenced. Amino acid variation was analyzed between the strain and all 11 reference sequences of GI.3 type retrieved from GenBank. Among the proteins encoded by ORF1, NS1 was the region most prone to amino acid variation (5.88%, 4/68), followed by NS6-NS7 (3.74%, 25/668), NS5 (2.63%, 3/114), NS2 (2.34%, 6/256), NS3 (1.17%, 4/341), VP1 (0.88%, 5/565), and NS4 (0.73%, 2/274). In the VP2 region encoded by ORF2, 5.45% of amino acid variation was observed (9/165). The results are shown in Appendix A, Tables 5 and A2.

Table 5. Amino acid variation of ORF2 in genotype GI.3.

					VP2				
	31	**46**	**137**	**138**	**149**	**150**	**151**	**159**	**165**
SD20230757	A	T	S	A	N	T	G	S	V
LC504389		I	P					T	
LC504390	T		P					T	
LC504391			P						
LC504392			P	T				T	
LC504393		I	P					T	
LC504394		I	P					T	
LC504395		I	P				C	T	
AB623037			P					T	
AB522396		I	P		S				A
MG012401			P						A
PQ510869			P			I			

4. Discussion

Though studies on gastroenteritis viruses have mostly focused on norovirus and rotavirus, SaV is a key pathogen responsible for sporadic infection and outbreaks of acute gastroenteritis in humans [3]. In a study conducted in Japan by Hoque et al., the SaV positivity rate was 8.30% [8]. In a subsequent study by Li et al., the SaV positivity rate was

2.77% [13]. A separate study in Spain reported a SaV positivity rate of 8% [14]. Our study recorded a SaV positivity rate of 1.12% in Shandong during 2022–2023, which is relatively low compared to previous studies. Countries such as Japan, Spain, and Burkina Faso have incorporated the rotavirus vaccine into their national immunization programs, which likely contributes to the increasing prominence of their higher SaV positivity rates. In addition, this study covered the whole age group, while other studies mostly covered children, and our study also found that the positive rate in children aged 3–5 was significantly higher than that in other age groups. It is worth mentioning here that SaV can infect both preschool-aged children and the elderly. Young children, particularly those under the age of five, are highly susceptible due to their immature immune systems and frequent exposure to communal environments such as daycare centers. The SaV positivity rate in 2023 was significantly higher than that in 2022. In late 2022, changes in COVID-19 control strategies in Shandong Province may have contributed to an altered SaV epidemiological landscape in 2023, resulting in increased detection rates.

SaV was detected throughout the year, but in this study, no cases were reported in April 2022, possibly due to the severe precautionary measures because of the COVID-19 outbreak in Shandong Province from March to May 2022. In both 2022 and 2023, the highest SaV positivity rates were observed in November, consistent with the findings of Ji et al. [15]. This was earlier than the peaks observed by Hoque et al. and Li et al. [8,13]. But all studies showed the peaks occurred in cold months, aligning with the study by Dey et al. [16]. It is recommended that medical institutions adopt a more targeted testing approach.

This study examined the prevalence of SaV in 16 cities across Shandong Province during 2022–2023. The highest SaV positivity rate in 2022 was observed in Dongying City, which was explained by the effective control of COVID-19 that allowed for normal population movement. In addition, Zaozhuang City recorded the highest SaV positivity rate in 2023. This study also highlighted fluctuations in SaV positivity rates across different cities over time, emphasizing the importance of ongoing viral diarrhea surveillance to monitor long-term trends.

SaV infection is considered mild, but our study showed no significant difference in SaV positivity rates between outpatient and inpatient cases. The number of SaV-positive cases in this study was relatively low; therefore, expanded surveillance is required to better assess the severity of clinical symptoms. A comparison between SaV-positive and SaV-negative patients in this study revealed that vomiting was a distinctive symptom associated with SaV infection. This is consistent with the results of Tang et al. [17]. It is suggested that more attention be paid to vomiting symptoms in SaV surveillance in the future. SaV is characterized by diverse transmission modes, high viral shedding, and low infectious doses [18]. Proper handling of vomitus from SaV-infected patients is essential to prevent these materials from becoming risk factors for outbreaks, which could lead to significant public health concerns.

The adoption of a dual-typing method provides a more comprehensive understanding of SaV sequences [10]. In this study, a dual-typing method was used based on the VP1 and RdRp nucleotide sequences. The predominant genotype in Shandong was identified as GI.1[P1], which aligns with findings from several regions where GI.1 is also the dominant genotype [19–22]. Furthermore, this study identified three additional genotypes, i.e., GI.3, GII.1, and GIV.1 in 2023 compared to 2022, reflecting an increase in genotype diversity. The complete genome sequence of a GI.3 strain revealed that NS1 was the region most prone to amino acid variation, followed by VP2, which is consistent with the result for GI.1 SaV [23]. Considering that most of the current studies are on VP1, future studies should pay more attention to other regions, and SaV surveillance based on whole-genome sequencing is essential.

In summary, we studied 14,011 cases of gastroenteritis across all age groups during and after the COVID-19 epidemic. An upward trend and an increase in the genotype diversity of SaV were observed after the COVID-19 epidemic in our study. In addition, with the wider use of the rotavirus vaccine in Shandong, it is essential to conduct continuous surveillance on SaV.

Author Contributions: Conceptualization, Z.K., Z.F., M.G. and M.L.; methodology, Z.K., Z.F., M.G., M.L., T.L. and W.S.; software, Z.F., M.G., M.L. and K.D.; validation, Z.K., Z.F., T.L. and W.S.; formal analysis, M.G. and M.L.; investigation, M.G., M.L., K.D. and S.Y.; resources, Z.K. and Z.F.; data curation, Z.K., Z.F., M.G. and M.L.; writing—original draft preparation, M.G. and M.L.; writing—review and editing, Z.K., Z.F., M.G. and M.L.; visualization, M.G., M.L. and S.Y.; supervision, Z.K. and Z.F.; project administration, Z.K., Z.F., T.L. and W.S.; funding acquisition, Z.K. All authors have read and agreed to the published version of the manuscript.

Funding: This work was supported by the National Key Research and Development Program of China (2021YFC2302003).

Institutional Review Board Statement: We confirm that all methods were carried out in accordance with the Declaration of Helsinki and all experimental protocols were approved by the Ethics Committee of Shandong Provincial Center for Disease Control and Prevention (protocol code SDJK(K)2024-039-01).

Informed Consent Statement: Informed consent was obtained from all subjects involved in this study.

Data Availability Statement: The sequences obtained in this study are available at the NCBI GenBank repository with accession number PV014972.

Acknowledgments: We would like to thank all the reviewers for their valuable comments and suggestions to improve the quality of our article.

Conflicts of Interest: The authors declare no conflicts of interest.

Appendix A

Appendix A.1

Table A1. Genotype distribution by year.

Year	Genotype	Case (N)	Composition Ratio (%)	P-Genotype	Case (N)	Composition Ratio (%)	Dual Genotype	Case (N)	Composition Ratio (%)
2022	GI.1	8	30.77	GI.P1	7	35.00	GI.1[P1]	7	38.89
	GI.2	8	30.77	GI.P2	5	25.00	GI.2[P2]	4	22.22
	GI.6	1	3.85	GI.P6	1	5.00	GI.6[P6]	1	5.56
	GII.3	6	23.08	GII.P3	6	30.00	GII.3[P3]	5	27.78
	GII.5	3	11.54	GII.P5	1	5.00	GII.5[P5]	1	5.56
Total		26	100.00		20	100.00		18	100.00
2023	GI.1	20	31.25	GI.P1	18	37.50	GI.1[P1]	18	37.50
	GI.2	7	10.94	GI.P2	5	10.42	GI.2[P2]	5	10.42
	GI.3	2	3.13	GI.P3	2	4.17	GI.3[P3]	2	4.17
	GI.6	7	10.94	GI.P6	4	8.33	GI.6[P6]	4	8.33
	GII.1	10	15.63	GII.P1	10	20.83	GII.1[P1]	10	20.83
	GII.3	4	6.25	GII.P3	4	8.33	GII.3[P3]	4	8.33
	GII.5	11	17.19	GII.P5	3	6.25	GII.5[P5]	3	6.25
	GIV.1	3	4.69	GII.P10	2	4.17	GIV.1[GII.P10]	2	4.17
Total		64	100.00		48	100.00		48	100.00

Appendix A.2

Table A2. Amino acid variation of ORF1 in genotype GI.3.

		NS1				NS2					NS3			NS4			NS5						
	42	49	55	64	96	105	199	223	314	319	375	409	560	642	700	932	983	1044	1052	1096	1111	1123	1129	1204
SD20230757	F	S	A	R	A	T	T	E	I	S	I	E	S	N	S	S	D	A	E	P	T	D	F	T
LC504389		G	V							T						T					A	G		
LC504390																T					A	G		
LC504391																					A	E		
LC504392					T											T	E				A	E		A
LC504393	S		V							T						T					A	G		
LC504394		G	V							T						T					A	G		
LC504395		G	V							T						T		V			A	G		
AB623037																T					A	G		
AB522396	L		V	K	T	A		D			V	D			N	T					A	E	Y	
MG012401	S				P	A								T		T			A	S	A	E		
PQ510869			I				T		V				S											

								NS6-NS7															VP1		
	1205	1207	1221	1243	1305	1340	1342	1353	1362	1367	1400	1440	1490	1514	1533	1573	1588	1607	1635	1646	1735	1944	1994	1997	2232
SD20230757	V	S	I	P	R	E	I	D	V	A	V	T	I	I	E	G	D	P	A	S	T	K	A	V	V
LC504389							A							V				A	T					I	
LC504390	I						A							V				A	T						
LC504391																		A							
LC504392							A							V				A	T	G					
LC504393							A							V				A	T					I	
LC504394							A							V				A	T					I	
LC504395							A							V				A	T					I	
AB623037							A							V				A	T						
AB522396					K	D	T				I			V	D	S		A	T		I	R			
MG012401		N	V		K		T	E	I	V			V	V		S	E	A	T				S		I
PQ510869				S								A													

References

1. Madeley, C.R.; Cosgrove, B.P. Letter: Caliciviruses in man. *Lancet* **1976**, *1*, 199–200. [CrossRef] [PubMed]
2. Rockx, B.; De Wit, M.; Vennema, H.; Vinje, J.; De Bruin, E.; Van Duynhoven, Y.; Koopmans, M. Natural history of human calicivirus infection: A prospective cohort study. *Clin. Infect. Dis.* **2002**, *35*, 246–253. [CrossRef]
3. Oka, T.; Wang, Q.; Katayama, K.; Saif, L.J. Comprehensive review of human sapoviruses. *Clin. Microbiol. Rev.* **2015**, *28*, 32–53. [CrossRef]
4. Moraes, M.T.B.; Leitao, G.A.A.; Olivares, A.I.O.; Xavier, M.; Bispo, R.S.; Sharma, S.; Leite, J.P.G.; Svensson, L.; Nordgren, J. Molecular Epidemiology of Sapovirus in Children Living in the Northwest Amazon Region. *Pathogens* **2021**, *10*, 965. [CrossRef] [PubMed]
5. Becker-Dreps, S.; Gonzalez, F.; Bucardo, F. Sapovirus: An emerging cause of childhood diarrhea. *Curr. Opin. Infect. Dis.* **2020**, *33*, 388–397. [CrossRef]
6. Jiao, Y.; Han, T.; Qi, X.; Gao, Y.; Zhao, J.; Zhang, Y.; Li, B.; Zhang, Z.; Du, J.; Sun, L. Genotypes Diversity of Acute Gastroenteritis Outbreaks Caused by Human Sapovirus—Beijing Municipality, China, 2015-2021. *China CDC Wkly.* **2023**, *5*, 625–631. [CrossRef] [PubMed]
7. Cho, S.R.; Yun, S.J.; Chae, S.J.; Jung, S.; Kim, J.H.; Yong, K.C.; Cho, E.H.; Choi, W.; Lee, D.Y. An Outbreak Associated with Sapovirus GI.3 in an Elementary School in Gyeonggi-do, Korea. *J. Korean Med. Sci.* **2020**, *35*, e281. [CrossRef]
8. Hoque, S.A.; Pham, N.T.K.; Onda-Shimizu, Y.; Nishimura, S.; Sugita, K.; Kobayashi, M.; Islam, M.T.; Okitsu, S.; Khamrin, P.; Maneekarn, N.; et al. Sapovirus infections in Japan before and after the emergence of the COVID-19 pandemic: An alarming update. *J. Med. Virol.* **2023**, *95*, e29023. [CrossRef]
9. Traore, K.A.; Akapovi, M.M.; Ouedraogo, N.; Ouoba, J.B.; Roques, P.; Barro, N. Geographical distribution of enteric pathogenic viruses in Burkina Faso: A systematic review and meta-analysis. *BMC Infect. Dis.* **2024**, *24*, 756. [CrossRef]
10. Zhao, W.; Gao, Z.; Guo, C.; Zhang, Y.; Zhang, Y.; Wang, Q.; Yu, J. A dual typing system establishment and global diversity analysis for sapoviruses. *BMC Genom.* **2024**, *25*, 1131. [CrossRef]
11. Hall, T.A. BioEdit: A user-friendly biological sequence alignment editor and analysis program for Windows 95/98/NT. *Nucleic Acids Symp. Ser.* **1999**, *41*, 95–98.
12. Kumar, S.; Stecher, G.; Li, M.; Knyaz, C.; Tamura, K. MEGA X: Molecular Evolutionary Genetics Analysis across Computing Platforms. *Mol. Biol. Evol.* **2018**, *35*, 1547–1549. [CrossRef] [PubMed]
13. Li, S.; Yan, H.; Gao, Z.; Tian, Y.; Li, W.; Shen, L.; Liu, B.; Jia, L.; Wang, Q.; He, Y. Infection characteristics of sapoviruses in diarrhea cases admitted to the intestinal clinics in 2019, Beijing. *Int. J. Virol.* **2021**, *28*, 222–225. [CrossRef]
14. de Oliveira-Tozetto, S.; Santiso-Bellon, C.; Ferrer-Chirivella, J.M.; Navarro-Lleo, N.; Vila-Vicent, S.; Rodriguez-Diaz, J.; Buesa, J. Epidemiological and Genetic Characterization of Sapovirus in Patients with Acute Gastroenteritis in Valencia (Spain). *Viruses* **2021**, *13*, 184. [CrossRef]
15. Ji, X.; Guo, C.; Dai, Y.; Chen, L.; Chen, Y.; Wang, S.; Sun, Y. Genomic Characterization and Molecular Evolution of Sapovirus in Children under 5 Years of Age. *Viruses* **2024**, *16*, 146. [CrossRef]
16. Dey, S.K.; Phathammavong, O.; Nguyen, T.D.; Thongprachum, A.; Chan-It, W.; Okitsu, S.; Mizuguchi, M.; Ushijima, H. Seasonal pattern and genotype distribution of sapovirus infection in Japan, 2003–2009. *Epidemiol. Infect.* **2012**, *140*, 74–77. [CrossRef]
17. Tang, X.; Hu, Y.; Zhong, X.; Xu, H. Molecular Epidemiology of Human Adenovirus, Astrovirus, and Sapovirus Among Outpatient Children With Acute Diarrhea in Chongqing, China, 2017-2019. *Front. Pediatr.* **2022**, *10*, 826600. [CrossRef] [PubMed]
18. Becker-Dreps, S.; Bucardo, F.; Vinje, J. Sapovirus: An important cause of acute gastroenteritis in children. *Lancet Child Adolesc. Health* **2019**, *3*, 758–759. [CrossRef]
19. Doan, Y.H.; Yamashita, Y.; Shinomiya, H.; Motoya, T.; Sakon, N.; Suzuki, R.; Shimizu, H.; Shigemoto, N.; Harada, S.; Yahiro, S.; et al. Distribution of Human Sapovirus Strain Genotypes over the Last Four Decades in Japan: A Global Perspective. *Jpn J. Infect. Dis.* **2023**, *76*, 255–258. [CrossRef]
20. Zhuo, R.; Ding, X.; Freedman, S.B.; Lee, B.E.; Ali, S.; Luong, J.; Xie, J.; Chui, L.; Wu, Y.; Pang, X.; et al. Molecular Epidemiology of Human Sapovirus among Children with Acute Gastroenteritis in Western Canada. *J. Clin. Microbiol.* **2021**, *59*, e0098621. [CrossRef]
21. Phengma, P.; Khamrin, P.; Jampanil, N.; Yodmeeklin, A.; Ukarapol, N.; Maneekarn, N.; Kumthip, K. Molecular epidemiology and characterization of norovirus and sapovirus in pediatric patients with acute diarrhea in Thailand, 2019–2020. *J. Infect. Public Health* **2022**, *15*, 1013–1019. [CrossRef] [PubMed]
22. Mann, P.; Pietsch, C.; Liebert, U.G. Genetic Diversity of Sapoviruses among Inpatients in Germany, 2008–2018. *Viruses* **2019**, *11*, 726. [CrossRef] [PubMed]
23. Hoque, S.A.; Akari, Y.; Khamrin, P.; Phan, T.; Onda, Y.; Okitsu, S.; Komoto, S.; Hayakawa, S.; Komine-Aizawa, S.; Yuki, Y.; et al. Epidemiology and molecular evolution of GI.1 sapovirus in the recent era. *J. Med. Virol.* **2024**, *96*, e29904. [CrossRef] [PubMed]

viruses

MDPI

Article

Molecular Epidemiology of Human Adenovirus from Acute Gastroenteritis Cases in Brazil After the COVID-19 Pandemic Period, 2021–2023

Mateus de Souza Mello, Fábio Correia Malta, Alexandre Madi Fialho, Fernanda Marcicano Burlandy and Tulio Machado Fumian *

Laboratório de Virologia Comparada e Ambiental, Instituto Oswaldo Cruz (IOC), Fundação Oswaldo Cruz (FIOCRUZ), Rio de Janeiro CEP 21045-900, Brazil; mello.souza.mateus@gmail.com (M.d.S.M.); fabio.malta@ioc.fiocruz.br (F.C.M.); amfialho@ioc.fiocruz.br (A.M.F.); fburlandy@ioc.fiocruz.br (F.M.B.)
* Correspondence: tuliomf@ioc.fiocruz.br or fumiantm@gmail.com

Abstract: Human enteric adenoviruses (HAdV-F40/41) play a crucial role as causative agents of acute gastroenteritis (AGE), particularly affecting children in low-and middle-income countries. This study investigated the prevalence, genetic diversity, and molecular characteristics of HAdV-F40/41 in AGE cases reported in Brazil from 2021 to 2023, a period after the COVID-19 pandemic. A total of 1980 stool samples collected from medically attended AGE patients from nine states were analyzed by TaqMan-based qPCR. Overall, HAdV was detected in 16.6% (*n* = 328/1980) of cases, with the highest prevalence observed in children under five years of age. The positive HAdV samples were genotyped through partial sequencing of the hexon and/or fiber genes followed by phylogenetic analysis. Enteric HAdVs (HAdV-F40/41) were detected in 3.2% (*n* = 63/1980) of samples, with HAdV-F41 (44.1%) being the most common genotype. Among the non-enteric types, HAdV-C (29.4%) was the most prevalent, followed by HAdV-B (13.2%), HAdV-A (10.3%), and HAdV-D (2.9%). Phylogenetic analysis of the hexon (HVR1–HVR6) and fiber (Shaft) gene regions identified two major clusters, H-GTC1 and F-GTC2, showing close genetic relationships with global strains. HAdV-F40/41 demonstrated significantly higher viral loads compared to non-enteric HAdVs. These findings highlight the importance of continued surveillance of HAdV-F to better understand its role in AGE cases and support public health strategies, including potential vaccine development.

Keywords: human adenovirus (HAdV); acute gastroenteritis (AGE); molecular epidemiology; HAdV-F40/41

1. Introduction

Acute gastroenteritis (AGE) is a leading cause of death worldwide, particularly in low-and middle-income countries (LMICs) [1,2]. It accounts for approximately 1.7 billion cases and 1.1 million deaths annually worldwide, primarily affecting children under 5 years of age in LMICs [3,4]. Among the viral agents related to AGE, the most common viruses involved in epidemic cases and outbreaks include rotavirus, norovirus, human adenovirus (HAdV), astrovirus, and sapovirus [5,6]. According to the International Committee on the Taxonomy of Viruses (ICTV), HAdVs belong to the *Adenoviridae* family, within the *Mastadenovirus* genus (ICTV; https://ictv.global/, accessed on 15 January 2025) [7]. They are non enveloped viruses that comprise a linear double-stranded DNA genome measuring approximately 35 kb in size, containing multiple open reading frames (ORFs) that encode

 https://doi.org/10.3390/v17040577

proteins with different functions [8–10]. The structure of the viral capsid is icosahedral and can be classified into three distinct groups: major capsid proteins (hexon, penton base, and fiber), minor proteins (IIIa, VI, VIII, and IX) and non-structural proteins (IVa2, V, VII, μ, terminal, and protease) [11].

HAdVs are divided into seven different species (A–G), and 116 distinct genotypes have been identified using molecular methodologies (http://hadvwg.gmu.edu/, accessed on 15 January 2025) [12,13]. The symptomatic profile of each HAdV varies depending mainly on intrinsic factors (tropism and receptor affinity) such as viral extrinsic factors (age and immunodeficiency of the individual) [14–18]. These viruses can be responsible for manifestations associated with the respiratory, gastrointestinal, and ocular tracts, in addition to rare infections of the urinary tract, hepatocytes, and nerve cells [19]. While immunocompetent individuals tend to develop a self-limiting condition, immunosuppression patients, such as transplant recipients, tend to have a more complex development of the pathology [20–22]. Genotypes 40 and 41, within the F species (also known as enteric adenoviruses), have been well recognized as important cause of AGE, primarily affecting children under 5 years of age and accounting for around 3% to 12% of infantile AGE cases [23–27].

Cohen et al. [28], who have worked in LMICs, have identified HAdV-F40/41 as the second most frequently detected pathogen in children under five years of age with AGE, behind only rotaviruses [28]. A study on HAdV-F41 in children younger than six years old has identified distinct mutation profiles, with the short fiber region demonstrating greater permissiveness to these genetic changes [29]. A 10-year study conducted in Kenya investigating HAdV genetic diversity in children under 13 years old identified five HAdV-F40 and seven HAdV-F41 clades, highlighting previously unrecognized viral heterogeneity in the region [30]. A recent study performed in England during the COVID-19 pandemic demonstrated a difference in the prevalence of lineages and the predominance of the 2b lineage [31].

In Brazil, the rotavirus vaccine (RV1, Rotarix) was incorporated into the National Immunization Program in 2006, resulting in a significant reduction in RVA-related infections, hospitalizations, and deaths [32]. In previous studies from our group, we demonstrated an increase in noroviruses and HAdV circulation post-rotavirus vaccine introduction, showing these agents as a major cause of AGE in Brazil [33,34]. Few studies have been carried out to elucidate either the epidemiology or genetic diversity of HAdV-F40/41 [35–37]. In a previous study conducted by our group, HAdV was detected in 24.5% of AGE cases in Brazil between 2018 and 2020 [33]. Additionally, during the COVID-19 pandemic, cases of severe acute hepatitis of unknown etiology were reported in the United States and Ireland; some cases were linked to HAdV-F41 infections, highlighting the importance of HAdV surveillance at the country level [38,39]. Therefore, our study aimed to investigate the circulation, prevalence, and molecular diversity of HAdV during a three-year period (2021–2023) in AGE cases in Brazil. We also explored the genetic variability of enteric HAdV-F40/41 by sequencing the six hypervariable regions from the hexon gene (HVR1–HVR6), as well as the shaft in the long-fiber region.

2. Materials and Methods

2.1. Stool Samples and Ethical Aspects

Over three years, between January 2021 and December 2023, this study analyzed 1980 stool samples from medically attended patients (both children and adults) with AGE symptoms from nine states across the Southern, Southeastern, and Northeastern regions of Brazil. AGE was characterized by the sudden onset of diarrhea, with at least three liquid or semi-liquid stools within a 24 h period, with or without fever and vomiting. Stool samples were collected from clinically attended patients with AGE, together with clinical–epidemiological data. Samples were forwarded to the Laboratory of Comparative and Environmental Virology, which houses the Regional Reference Laboratory for Rotavirus (RRRL) at the Oswaldo Cruz Institute, Fiocruz, and were kept frozen at −20 °C until use. The RRRL is part of the national rotavirus surveillance program, under the supervision of the General Coordination of Public Health Laboratories of the Brazilian Ministry of Health.

This study is currently approved by the Ethics Committee of the Oswaldo Cruz Foundation (FIOCRUZ), Brazil (Approval number: CAAE: 76063123.5.0000.5248), and conducted according to the guidelines of the Declaration of Helsinki. Stool samples were manipulated anonymously, and patient data were maintained securely in compliance with the Ethical Protocol Statement ABNT NBR ISO 15189:2015. Patient-informed consent was waived by the Fiocruz Ethical Committee, and patients' data were maintained anonymously and securely.

2.2. *Viral Nucleic Acid Extraction*

Viral nucleic acids were extracted from 140 μL of clarified stool suspension (10% *w/v*) using Tris-calcium buffer (pH = 7.2). Samples underwent an automated nucleic acid extraction process utilizing the QIAcube® automated system and the QIAamp Viral RNA Mini Kit (both from QIAGEN, Valencia, CA, USA), in accordance with the manufacturer's guidelines. Nucleic acids were eluted using 60 μL of the elution buffer AVE and were promptly stored at −80 °C prior to molecular analysis. In every extraction procedure, RNAse/DNAse-free water served as the negative control.

2.3. *HAdV Detection and Quantification*

A multiplex TaqMan-based quantitative PCR (qPCR) method was employed for detection and quantification of all HAdV types and specifically the enteric F types. The multiplex qPCR combined a degenerate set of primers and a probe targeting a conserved region of the hexon gene to detect all HAdV types, in addition to primers and a probe used specifically for HAdV-F targeting the fiber region [40,41]. Detailed information on initial HAdV detection and quantification methods has been previously described [42]. Briefly, multiplex qPCR reactions were performed with 5 μL of the extracted DNA in a final volume of 20 μL, containing 10 μL of the 2× QuantiTect Probe PCR Kit (Qiagen, Valencia, CA, USA) and primers and probes with final concentrations of 1 μM and 0.25 μM, respectively. Reactions were conducted in the Applied Biosystems 7500 Real-Time PCR System (Applied Biosystems, Foster City, CA, USA) under the following thermal cycling conditions: 2 min at 50 °C, 15 min at 95 °C, 40 cycles of 15 s at 95 °C, and 1 min at 60 °C. Samples that exhibited a characteristic sigmoid curve and crossed the threshold line with a cycle threshold (Ct) value < 40 were considered positive. All runs included negative and positive controls (stool sample), as well as a non-template control. This study used all the rotavirus-and norovirus-negative samples (n = 1590), and additionally, HAdV was tested in ~35% of the positive samples for rotavirus and norovirus (n = 390).

2.4. *Rotavirus and Norovirus Detection*

Rotavirus and norovirus were identified and quantified using TaqMan-based RT-qPCR protocols. For rotavirus, primers (NSP3F and R) and a probe (NSP3p) were used to amplify the conserved NSP3 gene. For the detection of noroviruses GI and GII, it was used primer pairs (COG1F and R; COG2F and R) and probes (RING1C and RING2) targeted the ORF1/2 junction region, respectively [43,44].

2.5. HAdV Molecular Characterization and Genotyping

Conventional PCR was performed for the hexon protein using the primers Ad1 and Ad2, with an expected product of between 605 and 629 bp [45]. The reaction was carried out using 5 μL of extracted viral DNA and the 5× QIAGEN OneStep RT-PCR kit (Qiagen, Valencia, CA, USA), with primers at a final concentration of 0.2 μM. The reaction was performed under the following conditions: 1 holding step of 15 min at 95 °C followed by 40 cycles containing 1 min of denaturation at 95 °C, 1 min of annealing at 50 °C, and 1 min of extension at 72 °C. After 40 cycles, a final extension step at 72 °C was performed for 10 min. The PCR products were stored at −20 °C until the purification step.

For HAdV-F strains, we targeted the six hypervariable regions (HVR1–HVR6) of the hexon gene using the primers S29 and S52 and the partial shaft region of the long fiber gene using the primers AdF1 and AdF2 [46,47]. The PCR reactions were performed using the Platinum Taq DNA Polymerase enzyme (Invitrogen, Carlsbad, CA, USA), with 5 μL of extracted DNA in a final reaction volume of 25 μL. The expected amplicons for HAdV-F types 40 and 41 were 640 and 664 nt for the hexon gene and 508 and 530 nt for the fiber gene. All the amplicons were purified using the QIAquick Gel Extraction Kit (Qiagen, Hilden, Germany), following the manufacturer's recommendations. Sequencing reactions of the purified amplicons were performed using the Big Dye Terminator v.3.1 Cycle Sequencing Ready Reaction Kit on an ABI Prism 3730xl Genetic Analyzer (Applied Biosystems, Foster City, CA, USA) at the Fiocruz Institutional Genomic Platform for DNA sequencing (PDTIS).

2.6. Phylogenetic Analysis

HAdV chromatogram and consensus sequence analyses were performed using Geneious Prime 2021.1.1 (Biomatters Ltd., Auckland, New Zealand). For HAdV species and type assignment, an initial sequence analysis was performed using the Basic Local Alignment Search Tool (BLAST, accessed on 5 October 2024). HAdV reference sequences were obtained from the National Center for Biotechnology Information (NCBI) GenBank database and its outgroup; all sequences were aligned using MAFFT [48,49]. Phylogenetic trees of the partial hexon gene were constructed using the maximum likelihood method and selected the best-fit evolutionary model from jModeltest 2.1.6 for the dataset using the Tamura-Nei (TN93) +G + I model in MEGA X v. 10.2.6 [50–52]. The phylogenetic reconstruction method used was the maximum likelihood (1000 bootstraps iterations). Reference sequences were obtained from the National Center for Biotechnology Information (NCBI) GenBank database. In addition, to investigate the genetic diversity of the Brazilian HAdV-F strains, synonymous and non-synonymous mutations in the sequenced portions of the hexon and fiber genes were compared for each gene with prototype strains obtained from the GenBank database.

HAdV-F40/41 reference sequences were obtained from the National Center for Biotechnology Information (NCBI) GenBank database and its outgroup, and all sequences were aligned using MAFFT [48,49]. Phylogenetic trees of the partial hexon and fiber gene were constructed using the maximum likelihood method and the best-fit evolutionary model from jmodeltest 2.1.6 was selected for the dataset using the Hasegawa–Kishino-Yano (HKY) model for the fiber gene and HKY + I for the hexon gene [50,52,53]. The phylogenetic reconstruction method used was the maximum likelihood (1000 bootstraps iterations). The nucleotide sequences obtained in this study were deposited in the GenBank database under the accession numbers PV344519-PV344574 and PV392539-PV392576.

2.7. Statistical Analysis

Statistical analyses were performed using GraphPad Prism software v.9.0.0 (GraphPad Software, San Diego, CA, USA). Mann–Whitney U tests were used to assess significant differences between HAdV detection rates, years of collecting samples, viral load values between single and co-detection, age groups, and types. Fisher's exact tests were used for analyzing categorical characteristics in contingency tables. For all analyses, a p-value $\leq$ 0.05 was statistically significant.

3. Results

3.1. Epidemiologic Features of HAdV

Between January 2021 and December 2023, a total of 1980 stool samples were evaluated, both from patients with negative results for rotavirus and norovirus (n = 1590) and from samples positive for those viruses (n = 390). Overall, we detected HAdV in 16.6% (328/1980) of samples. Among the rotavirus- and norovirus-negative and positive samples, HAdV was detected in 15.7% and 20.4%, respectively. Enteric types HAdV-F40/41 were detected in 3.2% (n = 63) of the stool samples.

HAdV detection rates varied from 13% (76/583) in 2021 to 20.1% (145/723) in 2023 (Table 1). An increasing detection of HAdV was observed over the three years, with a significantly higher prevalence observed in 2023 compared to 2021 (p = 0.0008) and 2022 (p = 0.0437). During the three-year period, HAdV was detected in almost all months, except April and June 2021. Monthly detection rates varied from 4.6% in July 2022 to 31.4% in December 2023, with the latter being the highest detection rate observed during the study period (Figure 1A).

Table 1. Number of tested and HAdV-positive stool samples identified through laboratory-based surveillance by year and states in Brazil from 2021 to 2023.

States	No. Stool Samples—Positive/Total (%)			
	2021	2022	2023	Total
Bahia	8/55 (14.5)	0/2	0/0	8/57 (14)
Paraíba	0/0	1/2	10/28 (35.7)	11/30 (36.7)
Pernambuco	5/9	14/100 (14)	18/94 (19.1)	37/203 (18.2)
Sergipe	0/1	2/2	3/6	5/9
Espírito Santo	3/22 (13.6)	5/87 (5.7)	0/5	8/114 (7)
Minas Gerais	4/41(9.8)	14/81 (17.3)	66/230 (28.7)	84/352 (23.9)
Rio de Janeiro	0/18	6/39 (15.4)	1/4	7/61 (11.5)
Rio Grande do Sul	33/332 (10)	44/241 (18.3)	33/125 (26.4)	110/698 (15.8)
Santa Catarina	23/105 (21.9)	21/120 (17.5)	14/231 (6)	58/456 (12.7)
Total	76/583 (13)	107/674 (15.9)	145/723 (20.1)	328/1980 (16.6)

Over the cumulative period from 2021 to 2023, HAdV prevalence ranged from 12.6% in January to 32.9% in December (Figure 1B). With regards to seasonality, the prevalence was higher in spring (17.8%) compared to fall (15.4%), winter (15.9%), and summer (16%), although no significant differences were observed between seasons. (Figure 1C). During surveillance, the northeast revealed a high prevalence of HAdV (20.4%) when compared to the southeast (18.8%) and the south (14.6%), of which the detection in the south was significantly lower than that observed for the other two regions (Table 2). In the southeastern region, HAdV detection rates in 2023 were significantly higher compared to both 2021 (p = 0.0002) and 2022 ($p \leq$ 0.0001). The detection rates per year are shown in Table 2.

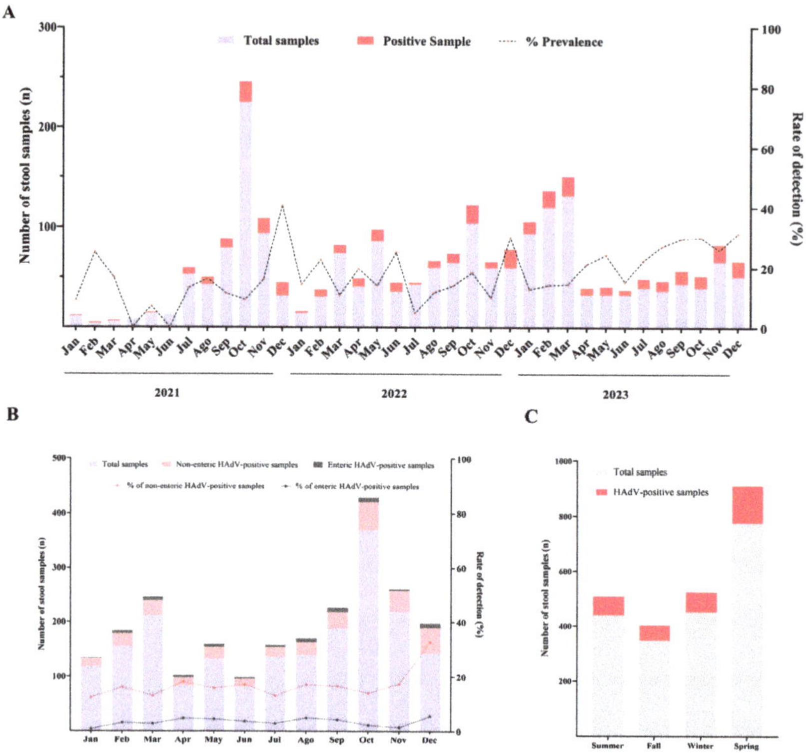

Figure 1. (**A**) Monthly distribution of tested acute gastroenteritis samples, HAdV-positive samples, and detection rates in Brazil, 2021–2023. (**B**) Monthly distribution of surveillance period addition of acute gastroenteritis samples tested. HAdV-positive samples and detection rates in Brazil. (**C**) Seasonal distribution period addition of HAdV-positive samples for each Brazilian region.

Table 2. Distribution of tested and HAdV-positive stool samples identified through laboratory-based surveillance by region in Brazil from 2021 to 2023.

Region	**No. of Stool Samples—Positive/Total (%)**				***p*-Value [a] (Fisher Test)**		
	2021	**2022**	**2023**	**Total**	**2021 vs. 2022**	**2021 vs. 2023**	**2022 vs. 2023**
Northeastern	13/65 (20)	17/106 (16)	31/128 (24.2)	61/299 (20.4)	0.5387	0.5880	0.1443
Southeastern	7/81 (8.6)	25/207 (12.1)	67/239 (28)	99/527 (18.8)	0.5323	0.0002	<0.0001
Southern	56/437 (12.8)	65/361 (18)	47/356 (13.2)	168/1154 (14.6)	0.0473	0.9156	0.0810
Total	76/583 (13)	107/674 (15.9)	145/723 (20.1)	328/1980 (16.6)	0.1728	0.0008	0.0437

[a] The *p*-values are indicated on the table (Fisher test).

The frequency of HAdV detection varied across age groups, ranging from 6.9% (57/823) in patients over 60 months to 24.7% (93/337) in children aged 12 to 24 months, and the detection rate was significantly higher among children up to 60 months old compared to older patients (Table 3).

Table 3. Number of tested and HAdV-positive fecal samples by age group in Brazil during 2021–2023.

Age Groups [a]	No. of Fecal Samples—Positive/Tested (%)			Total		*p*-Value [b]
	2021	2022	2023	All HAdV	HAdV-F	
0–12	16/91 (17.6)	22/101 (21.8)	39/156 (25)	77/348 (22.1)	14/348 (4)	<0.0001
12–24	20/110 (18.2)	29/132 (22)	44/135 (32.6)	93/377 (24.7)	17/377 (4.5)	<0.0001
24–60	25/133 (18.8)	41/157 (26.1)	35/142 (24.7)	101/432 (23.4)	23/432 (5.3)	<0.0001
>60	15/249 (6)	15/284 (5.3)	27/290 (9.3)	57/823 (6.9)	9/823 (1.1)	-

[a] age in months; [b] *p*-value < 0.0001 compared to all < 60 months. The *p*-values are indicated in the table (Fisher test).

3.2. Viral Load and Co-Detection Rates

The viral loads found in the samples ranged from 1.7×10^2 GC/g (genomic copies per gram of feces) to 2.3×10^{12} GC/g. When evaluating enteric and non-enteric HAdV, a significantly higher DNA load was observed in stool samples from patients positive for enteric HAdV compared to non-enteric strains (median of 1×10^8 vs. 1.2×10^4 GC/g, respectively) (Figure 2). With regard to age groups, we found a similar DNA viral load across the age groups analyzed, with median values varying from 5.8×10^3 GC/g in the group > 60 months to 6.4×10^4 GC/g in the age group of 24–60 months old.

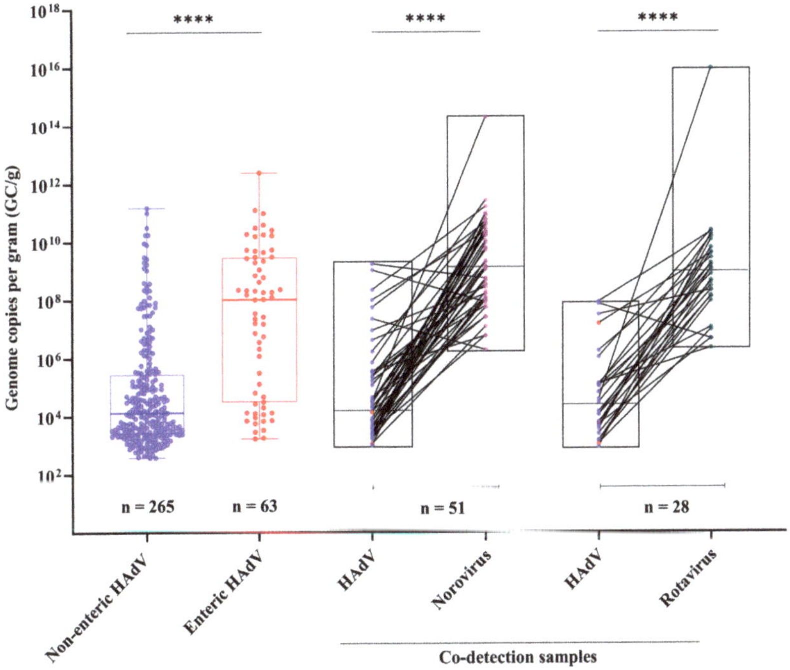

Figure 2. Distribution of viral load of non-enteric and enteric HAdV, noroviruses, and rotaviruses in stool samples, expressed as genome copies per gram (GC/g). Box-and-whisker plots show the first and third quartiles (equivalent to the 5th and 95th percentiles), the median (the horizontal line in the box). **** $p \leq 0.0001$.

In order to analyze the rate of co-detection of HAdV with rotavirus and norovirus, we selected around 30% of samples that previously tested positive for both viruses during the study period. Among rotavirus- and norovirus-positive samples, the HAdV detection rate was 24.1% (28/116), and 18.6% (51/274), respectively. Although HAdV was more frequently detected among rotavirus-positive samples, no significant difference was observed between the detection rates ($p = 0.2719$). Interestingly, among HAdV-positive samples that were co-infected with either rotavirus or norovirus, the level of HAdV DNA shedding was significantly lower ($p \leq 0.0001$) compared to the RNA load of the other viruses. Specifically, the median RNA load for rotavirus was 9.3×10^8 GC/g, and for norovirus it was also 1.4×10^{10} GC/g. In contrast, the median DNA load observed for HAdV was markedly lower, at 2.2×10^4 GC/g and 1.5×10^5 GC/g, respectively (Figure 2). Among the 79 HAdV-positive samples co-detected with rotavirus or norovirus, enteric and non-enteric HAdV were detected in seven (1.5%) and 73 (98.5%), respectively ($p \leq 0.0001$). The higher frequence of non-enteric HAdV in co-detected samples, in relatively low levels, may indicate a less active or secondary role in the infection.

3.3. Genetic Characterization HAdV

Among the HAdV analyzed, 20.7% (68/328) of samples collected between 2021 and 2023 were successfully sequenced. The obtained sequences were classified as species A, B, C, D, and F (Figure 3A), with HAdV-F being the most prevalent (44.1%). This species included genotypes F40 and F41, with HAdV-F41 being predominant across most age groups, showing a prevalence varying from 44% to 75% of the samples. In contrast, HAdV-F40 was identified at detection rates between 4% and 10.5%. An exception was observed in children aged between 12 and 24 months, where the prevalence of HAdV-F41 dropped to 15.8%. The second most frequent species was HAdV-C (29.4%), represented by genotypes C1, C2, and C5. Within this group, HAdV-C2 emerged as the dominant genotype in children aged >12–24 months (31.6%). The remaining species (A, B, and D) exhibited lower prevalence rates, ranging from 5% to 25% (Figure 3B). The complete quantitative distribution of HAdV strains is detailed in Figure 3C.

Among the non-enteric HAdV types, the most frequently detected genotype was HAdV-C2 ($n = 13$) (Figure 4). These isolates exhibited high genetic identity (98.3–100%) and were resolved into two distinct clusters with robust statistical support (99% bootstrap), suggesting potential intragenotypic variation. HAdV-B3 was the second most prevalent genotype ($n = 9$), with strains exhibiting 100% nucleotide identity among the Brazilian samples analyzed. The strains were closely related to a Germany strain (OR487155), demonstrating 99.4% of nucleotide identity. HAdV-A31, the third most detected genotype ($n = 6$), exhibited the highest intragenotypic divergence. Notably, one isolate (BRA/LVCA35542/2023/HAdV-31) showed reduced identity (95.5%) compared to others HAdV-A31 strains, highlighting potential evolutionary or geographic distinctions (Figure 4).

3.4. Diversity of Enteric HAdV

We characterized partial regions of the hexon and fiber genes from enteric HAdV-F40/41. A total of 28 samples were sequenced for the HVR1-HVR6 hexon region, and 30 samples were sequenced for the shaft of the fiber gene. During the study period, HAdV-F41 was the predominant genotype, detected in 86.7% ($n = 26$) of the samples, while HAdV-F40 was identified in 13.3% ($n = 4$). Regarding HAdV-F40, two samples identified from the fiber region were not represented in the phylogenetic reconstruction.

The phylogenetic analysis of the hexon region (HVR1-HVR6) of the Brazilian HAdV-F41 lineages revealed the presence of two lineages, H-GTC 1 and H-GTC 2 (Figure 5A), of which the majority of samples ($n = 21$) were identified within the H-GTC 1, while six samples were characterized as H-GTC 2. A high nt identity for the Brazilian isolates was observed in Cluster HGTC 1 (99.1–100%), with strains from Brazil (OQ442280 and OQ442288), India (MT952508), France (MW567963), Germany (ON442330), South Africa

(MK962806), Japan (LC790284, AB610523 and LC790290), China (PP844976, KY316160, KY316162 and MH465394), and the prototype strain TAK (DQ315364).

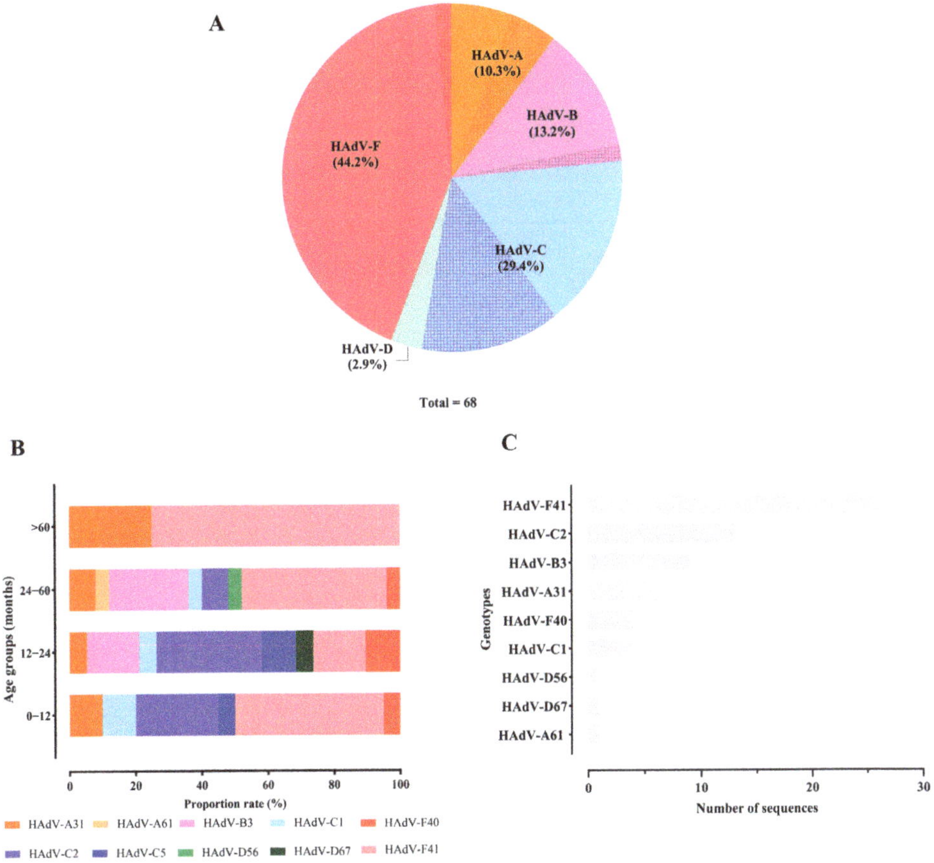

Figure 3. (**A**) The total frequency of HAdV types obtained from samples sequenced between 2021 and 2023. HAdV types obtained from co-detection with rotavirus or norovirus are represented by a hatched pattern. (**B**) Frequency by age group. (**C**) Distribution of HAdV genotypes identified in samples from Brazil between 2021 and 2023.

A high nt identity (>99% identity) was observed between samples from cluster H-GTC 2 and sequences from the United States (KF303069), Brazil (OQ442277, OQ442282 and OQ442296), and India (MT952501). The nucleotide (nt) identity between sequences HGTC 1 and HGTC 2 was 96.3%.

The HAdV-F40 genotype identified in this study exhibited a high nt identity, varying from 99.3% to 100%, with Brazilian isolates (OQ442264 and OQ442267), the prototype strain Dungan (L19443), and sequences reported from South Africa (MK955319) and India (MT952448). The high genetic conservation between geographically distinct HAdV-F40 strains reveals high conservation in the HVR region.

With regards to the HAdV-F40 strains, two samples had a 100% nt identity between them, and showed the highest nt similarity (ranging from 99–100%) with F40 sequences isolated in Brazil in 2018 to 2019 (OQ442231 and OQ442228), with sequences from India (MT952560), and with the prototype F40 strain Dungan (L19443). Pairwise comparison of nt sequences revealed a range of 95.7–96.5% sequence identity between HAdV-F40 and HAdV-F41 strains.

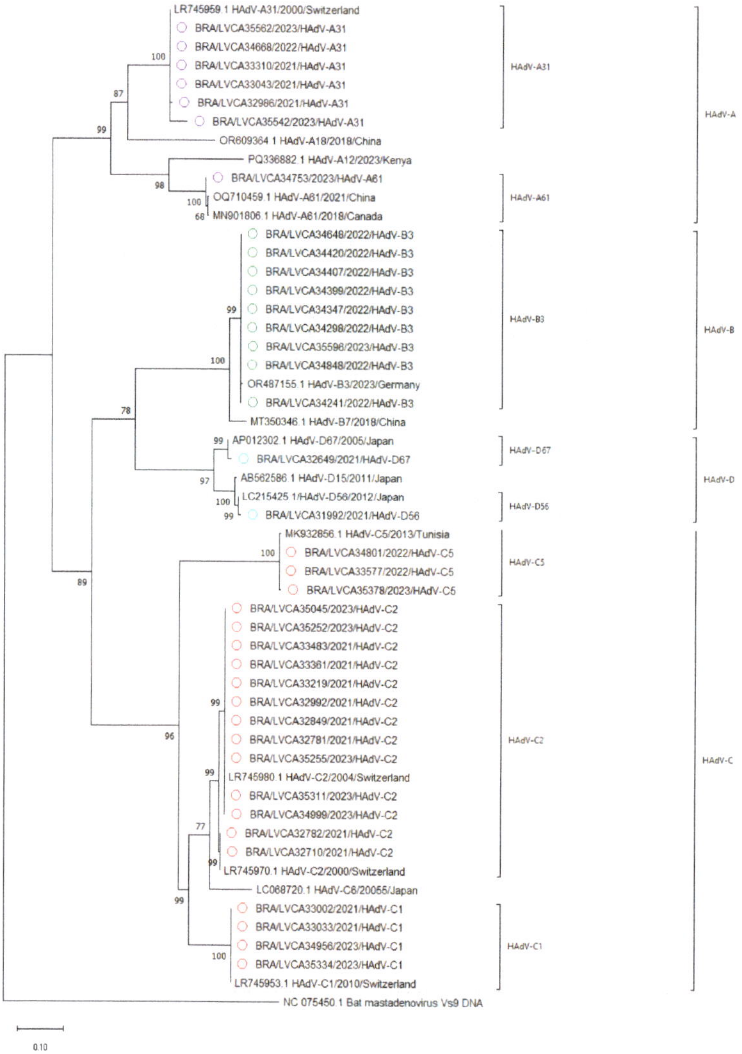

Figure 4. Phylogenetic tree based of non-enteric HAdV on the conserved region of the nucleotide (nt) sequences of the hexon gene. Strains isolated in this study (marked with a circle) are shown as country, LVCA internal register number, year of collection, and type (i.e., BRA/LVCA35334/2023/HAdV-C1) and Reference strains were downloaded from GenBank. Maximum likelihood phylogenetic trees were constructed using MEGA X software with bootstrap testing (1000 replicates) applied the on Tamura-Nei (TN93) +G + I. Bootstrap values above 60% are given at branch nodes.

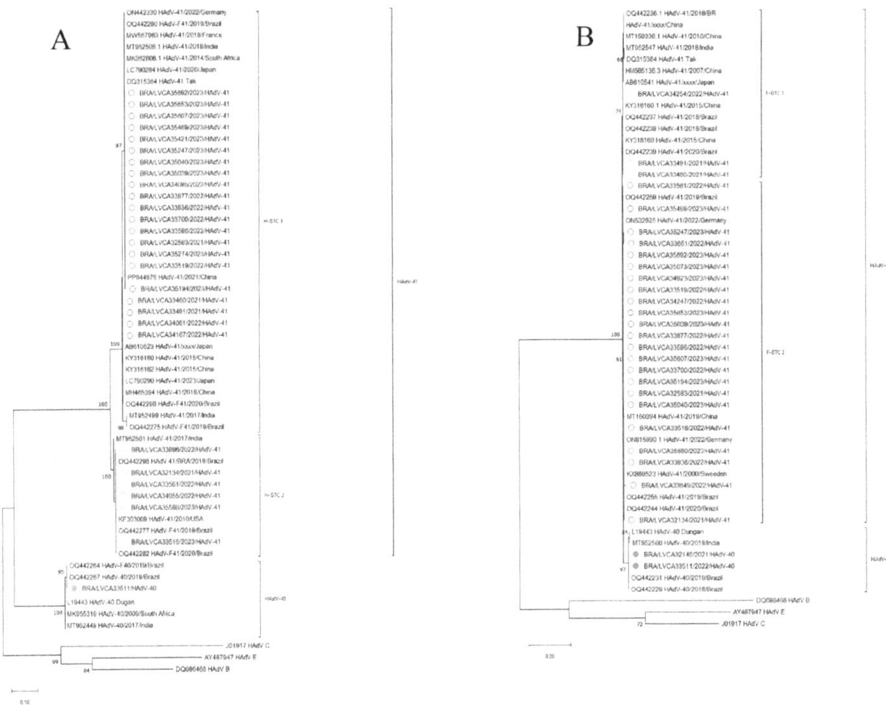

Figure 5. Phylogenetic tree based on the nt sequence of the (**A**) hypervariable regions (HVR1–HVR6) of the hexon gene and (**B**) partial shaft region of the fiber gene. HAdV-F40 and -F41. Strains isolated in this study (marked with a circle) are shown as country, LVCA internal register number, year of collection, and type (i.e., BRA/LVCA33516/2023/HAdV-41) and Reference strains were downloaded from GenBank. Maximum likelihood phylogenetic trees were constructed using MEGA X software with bootstrap testing (1000 replicates), applying the HKY model for the hexon hypervariable regions (**A**) and the HKY + I model for the fiber shaft region (**B**). Bootstrap values ≥ 60% are shown at branch nodes.

Phylogenetic analysis of the shaft region in the fiber gene revealed two distinct lineages within HAdV-F41: F-GTC 1 and F-GTC 2 (Figure 5B). Among the analyzed samples, 23 were classified under the F-GTC 2 lineage, while three belonged to the F-GTC 1 lineage. A high nt similarity (99.8%) was observed between the two clusters of HAdV-F41 strains. Our Brazilian strains of the cluster F-GTC 1 samples showed the highest nt similarity (100%) with samples from Japan (AB610541 and AB610541), China (AB610538, MT150336, HM565136 and KY316160), India (MT952547), and Brazil (OQ442236, OQ442237, OQ442238 and OQ442239). Samples within the cluster F-GTC 2 showed high nt similarity (99.8–100%) with samples from Germany (ON532825 and ON815890), Sweden (KX868523), Brazil (OQ442259, OQ442255, and OQ442244), and China (MT150394). The identity between group F-GTC 1 and F-GTC 2 ranged from 98.1% to 99.2%

4. Discussion

Our study provides insights into the prevalence, epidemiological features, and genetic diversity of HAdV among AGE cases in medically attended patients (symptomatic children and adults) across nine Brazilian states during the COVID-19 pandemic (2021–2023). During the study period, we detected HAdV at a prevalence rate of 16.6%. HAdV-F41 was the most prevalent genotype and accounted for more than 38.2% of total infections. Although multiple HAdV species were detected, the enteric types demonstrated significantly higher viral DNA shedding compared to non-enteric types. We also identified the enteric genotype HAdV-F41 as the predominant strain, accounting for most of the identified cases.

Globally, the prevalence of HAdV varies significantly, ranging from 2% to 39%, with the highest detection rates observed in low- and lower-middle-income countries [54–58]. Limited access to clean water, inadequate sanitation infrastructure, and higher population density, usually observed in LMICs, are likely key factors contributing to discrepancies [59,60]. In Brazil, studies conducted up to 2017 reported a prevalence of HAdV among AGE cases ranging from 4% to 7% [36,58,61]. Between 2018 and 2020, Do Nascimento et al. [33] found an overall prevalence of HAdV of 24.5% in eleven Brazilian states. In another two studies conducted in Brazil, HAdV was detected at prevalence rates of 28.6% and 18.5% in the Southeastern and Amazon regions, respectively [62,63].

In our study, we observed a decline in HAdV circulation in Brazil during the pandemic period, especially in the first semester of 2021, when the measures to control the spread of SARS-CoV-2 were stringent. These measures included the enforcement of social distancing, lockdowns, childcare and school closures, and mandatory use of face masking. Previous HAdV surveillance conducted by our group reported similar trends during the year of 2020. In that study, HAdV prevalence rates were 26.7% and 27.9% in 2018 and 2019, respectively, and decreased to 12.6% in 2020. During this study, similar prevalence rates (13% and 15.9%) were found in 2021 and 2022. In 2023, HAdV prevalence rebounded to 20.1%, returning to levels comparable to those observed in the pre-pandemic years [33]. Since the beginning of the COVID-19 pandemic, several studies reported a decrease in the circulation of several respiratory and enteric pathogens, especially viral infections in the pediatric population [64–68]. For instance, studies conducted in Norway, Thailand, Germany, and Poland demonstrated a reduction in the circulation of respiratory viruses (such as influenza virus A/B and rhinovirus) and gastroenteric viruses (HAdV, norovirus, and rotavirus), varying from 2% to 87% during the pandemic years [69–72]. Additionally, our findings align with data from studies conducted in China, Iraq, Albania, and India, between 2011 to 2017, which detected HAdV in over 20% of tested stool samples from children with AGE [73–76]. Two studies have identified HAdV as the primary and secondary leading pathogen responsible for diarrhea requiring hospitalization in India and Bangladesh, respectively [77,78].

Regarding age groups, we observed the highest prevalence of HAdV infections in children aged up to 60 months old. Studies conducted across several countries in Africa, Asia and Latin America on bacterial and viral pathogens have shown that enteric HAdV exhibit a higher attributable incidence in children under two years of age compared to those up to 5 years old, with rates ranging from 3.9 to 20.9 episodes of diarrhea per 100 child-years [79–81].

The HAdV co-detection rate found in rotavirus- and norovirus-positive was 20%. Interestingly, only 5.5% of these co-detected cases involved the enteric types F40/41. A significantly higher viral load of rotavirus and norovirus was observed compared to HAdV, suggesting that those viruses were likely the primary causative agent of AGE symptoms, rather than HAdV. A higher co-detection rate was previously reported by our group in samples from Brazil during the 2018–2020 period [33]. Co-detection between different enteric viruses and HAdV is not an uncommon report. Two retrospective studies conducted in India among pediatric patients have shown that HAdV was the main agent found in co-detection with norovirus [82,83]. In Brazil, during a norovirus-associated AGE outbreak in the Santa Catarina state, southern region, in 2023, HAdV was co-detected in 6.8% of norovirus-positive samples [84]. Similarly, studies conducted in the United States and

Canada have reported high rates of HAdV co-detection in AGE patients, with rates of 27% and 30.9%, respectively [85,86].

Overall, we found a higher predominance of enteric HAdV species (44.1%) compared to non-enteric species. Moreover, we demonstrated significantly higher viral DNA shedding in the group of F40/41-positive fecal samples. Given the ubiquitous nature of HAdV, with over 100 types capable of infecting humans and causing a wide range of clinical symptoms, including common conditions such as respiratory diseases and conjunctivitis, it is not surprising that non-enteric types were frequently detected [33,55,58,87–90].

During our study, we observed a significant predominance of HAdV-F41 (86.7%) compared to HAdV-F40 (13.3%) among the enteric types. Our data are similar to worldwide findings, revealing a global trend regarding HAdV genotype distribution among AGE cases [27,54,55,85,86]. In Brazil, during a surveillance study conducted in the same regions between 2018 and 2020, Nascimento et al., 2022 [33] observed that among HAdV-F species, type F41 was the most prevalent genotype (81.5%) [33]. This genotype was significantly more common than others, particularly among children under 24 months of age. In line with our data, other studies conducted in Brazil have reported similar findings, revealing that over 50% of the sequenced samples belonged to the HAdV-F41 genotype [35–37,58,91]. In Australia, a study using next-generation sequencing identified a pronounced predominance of serotype F41 (83.5%) among six major human adenovirus (HAdV) groups isolated from wastewater samples in Sydney and Melbourne, between 2016 and 2017 [92]. In this same study, clinical data further confirmed F41 as the predominant serotype, accounting for 52.5% of gastroenteritis cases, with C1 and C2 exhibiting lower prevalence rates [89]. In Venezuela, during a 13-year surveillance study conducted before and after the implementation of a rotavirus vaccine, HAdV was detected in 19.5% of AGE samples, with the domain (79.8%) of the genotype F41 [93]. More recently, a study conducted in India during the year of 2019 identified HAdV-F as the leading cause of AGE in children under 5 years of age, with a prevalence rate of 49.4% [94].

Phylogenetic analysis of the HVR region revealed that most Brazilian F41 strains grouped into the H-GTC1 cluster (n = 22), with a smaller proportion belonging to the H-GTC 2 lineage (n = 6). Only one sample was identified as HAdV-F40. These findings contrast with those of a previous study by our group, where the majority of the samples were classified as H-GTC 2 [42]. Studies carried out in Germany and India have also reported the co-circulation of multiple HAdV-F41 lineages, with lineage 2 being particularly prevalent [94,95]. Interestingly, over the six-year surveillance period, our group observed a shift in the circulation of these lineages in Brazil. The reason for this remains unclear, but the data suggest that immune pressure may have driven the genotype replacement.

From the shaft region, we observed a predominance of cluster F41-GTC 2 (n = 23) compared to F41-GTC 1 (n = 3). Only two samples were detected as HAdV-F40. These data are similar to those observed in Kenya, Brazil, and India [30,42,94]. Recent studies analyzing the complete genome of HAdV-F41 have identified the hexon and fiber (both short and long) genes, as well as the E3 and E4 regions, as the main sites of mutation within the HAdV genome [30,31,95].

During our study, among the non-enteric HAdV types, the most prevalent species was HAdV-C (52.6%), represented by genotypes C1 and C2, followed by HAdV-B3. Several studies have reported that non-enteric HAdV genotypes, frequently detected in AGE stool samples, primarily belong to species A, B, C, and D, with HAdV-C being the most common. However, these genotypes are typically associated with other diseases rather than AGE [20,96–98].

Our study has some limitations. Firstly, we did not access detailed clinical/epidemiological data from patients, which hindered our ability to track non-enteric HAdV cases with other possible clinical symptoms. Secondly, we did not investigate non-viral enteropathogens, such as bacteria and parasites, or other AGE-related viruses that may be involved in clinical cases of AGE. Moreover, our study did not include an asymptomatic group, which could help us to consider HAdV's involvement in clinical symptoms. Thirdly, it was not possible to sequence all HAdV-positive samples, given that many samples showed high Ct values (Ct > 32), indicating lower viral loads. Our evolutionary analysis of species F was based on partial parts of the hexon and long fiber genes rather than the complete genome. Finally, we believe that a portion of HAdV-positive samples may represent prolonged viral shedding after previous infections and may not contribute to AGE in all positive cases, especially in samples with co-viral findings, non-enteric types, and low viral loads.

5. Conclusions

In conclusion, we describe here the epidemiological and molecular features of HAdV in medically attended patients with AGE in Brazil. We assessed the viral shedding, age distribution, and genetic diversity of HAdV-F40/41 strains. After the COVID-19 pandemic period, from 2021 to 2023, we identified HAdV in 16.6% of samples. The surveillance and molecular epidemiology of HAdV are essential to assess the circulation patterns of both enteric and non-enteric types, as well as to identify potential emerging strains at the population level. Our data demonstrate that HAdV is an important cause of AGE and should be included in diagnostic protocols along with rotavirus and norovirus, which are routinely tested in AGE surveillance programs in Brazil and many other countries. Therefore, maintaining expanded national surveillance is crucial to support public health and monitor future trends and changes in HAdV epidemiology in Brazil.

Author Contributions: Conceptualization, M.d.S.M. and T.M.F.; methodology, M.d.S.M., F.C.M. and T.M.F.; formal analysis, M.d.S.M., F.C.M., A.M.F. and T.M.F.; investigation, M.d.S.M., F.C.M. and T.M.F.; writing—original draft preparation, M.d.S.M. and T.M.F.; writing—review and editing, M.d.S.M., F.C.M., F.M.B. and T.M.F.; supervision, T.M.F.; project administration, T.M.F.; funding acquisition, T.M.F. All authors have read and agreed to the published version of the manuscript.

Funding: This work was supported by The Brazilian National Council for Scientific and Technological Development (Conselho Nacional de Desenvolvimento Científico e Tecnológico—CNPq), FAPERJ—Fundação Carlos Chagas Filho de Amparo à Pesquisa do Estado do Rio de Janeiro, Processo SEI 260003/000530/2023 (Ref. Proc. No. 200.171/2023; Jovem Cientista do Nosso Estado", Fumian, T.M.), PAEF-3 and CNPq PROEP/IOC 441653/2024-3 from the Oswaldo Cruz Institute, Fiocruz. Further support was provided by CGLab, Brazilian Ministry of Health. Fumian, T.M. is a Productivity Fellowship Researcher from the "Conselho Nacional de Desenvolvimento Científico e Tecnológico—CNPq". This research study is under the scope of the activities of Fiocruz as a Collaborating Center of PAHO/WHO of Public and Environmental Health.

Institutional Review Board Statement: This study was approved by the Ethics Committee of the Oswaldo Cruz Foundation (FIOCRUZ), number CAAE: 76063123.5.0000.5248 (approval date: 20 February 2024).

Informed Consent Statement: Patient-informed consent was waived by the Fiocruz Ethical Committee, and patients' data were maintained anonymously and securely.

Data Availability Statement: The data that support the findings of this study are openly available in the GenBank database. The datasets generated and analyzed during the current study are available in the GenBank repository under the following accession numbers cited in the Materials and Methods. This study is registered in the Brazilian National System for Genetic Heritage and Associated Traditional Knowledge Management (No. A837EB6).

Acknowledgments: We would like to thank the LVCA team for their excellent technical assistance. We also would like to thank the State Central Laboratories staff members coordinated by the Coordenação Geral de Laboratórios de Saúde Pública (CGLab)—Brazilian Ministry of Health for collecting the samples and data.

Conflicts of Interest: The authors declare no conflicts of interest.

References

1. Kotloff, K.L.; Nataro, J.P.; Blackwelder, W.C.; Nasrin, D.; Farag, T.H.; Panchalingam, S.; Wu, Y.; Sow, S.O.; Sur, D.; Breiman, R.F.; et al. Burden and Aetiology of Diarrhoeal Disease in Infants and Young Children in Developing Countries (the Global Enteric Multicenter Study, GEMS): A Prospective, Case-Control Study. *Lancet* **2013**, *382*, 209–222. [CrossRef] [PubMed]
2. The Top 10 Causes of Death. Available online: https://www.who.int/news-room/fact-sheets/detail/the-top-10-causes-of-death (accessed on 30 December 2023).
3. Number of Under-Five Deaths—By Cause. Available online: https://platform.who.int/data/maternal-newborn-child-adolescent-ageing/indicator-explorer-new/MCA/number-of-under-five-deaths---by-cause (accessed on 25 March 2024).
4. World Health Organization Diarrhoeal Disease. Available online: https://www.who.int/news-room/fact-sheets/detail/diarrhoeal-disease (accessed on 22 March 2024).
5. Akdag, A.I.; Gupta, S.; Khan, N.; Upadhayay, A.; Ray, P. Epidemiology and Clinical Features of Rotavirus, Adenovirus, and Astrovirus Infections and Coinfections in Children with Acute Gastroenteritis Prior to Rotavirus Vaccine Introduction in Meerut, North India. *J. Med. Virol.* **2020**, *92*, 1102–1109. [CrossRef] [PubMed]
6. Flynn, T.G.; Olortegui, M.P.; Kosek, M.N. Viral Gastroenteritis. *Lancet* **2024**, *403*, 862–876. [CrossRef] [PubMed]
7. Benkő, M.; Aoki, K.; Arnberg, N.; Davison, A.J.; Echavarría, M.; Hess, M.; Jones, M.S.; Kaján, G.L.; Kajon, A.E.; Mittal, S.K.; et al. ICTV Virus Taxonomy Profile: Adenoviridae 2022: This Article Is Part of the ICTV Virus Taxonomy Profiles Collection. *J. Gen. Virol.* **2022**, *103*, 001721. [CrossRef]
8. Tousimis, A.J.; Hilleman, M.R. Electron Microscopy of Type 4 Adenovirus Strain RI-67. *Virology* **1957**, *4*, 499–508. [CrossRef]
9. Valentine, R.C.; Hopper, P.K. Polyhedral Shape of Adenovirus Particles as Shown by Electron Microscopy. *Nature* **1957**, *180*, 928. [CrossRef]
10. Davison, A.J.; Benkő, M.; Harrach, B. Genetic Content and Evolution of Adenoviruses. *J. Gen. Virol.* **2003**, *84*, 2895–2908. [CrossRef]
11. San Martín, C. Latest Insights on Adenovirus Structure and Assembly. *Viruses* **2012**, *4*, 847–877. [CrossRef]
12. Robinson, C.M.; Singh, G.; Lee, J.Y.; Dehghan, S.; Rajaiya, J.; Liu, E.B.; Yousuf, M.A.; Betensky, R.A.; Jones, M.S.; Dyer, D.W.; et al. Molecular Evolution of Human Adenoviruses. *Sci. Rep.* **2013**, *3*, 1812. [CrossRef]
13. Hashimoto, S.; Gonzalez, G.; Harada, S.; Oosako, H.; Hanaoka, N.; Hinokuma, R.; Fujimoto, T. Recombinant Type Human Mastadenovirus D85 Associated with Epidemic Keratoconjunctivitis since 2015 in Japan. *J. Med. Virol.* **2018**, *90*, 881–889. [CrossRef]
14. Roelvink, P.W.; Lizonova, A.; Lee, J.G.M.; Li, Y.; Bergelson, J.M.; Finberg, R.W.; Brough, D.E.; Kovesdi, I.; Wickham, T.J. The Coxsackievirus-Adenovirus Receptor Protein Can Function as a Cellular Attachment Protein for Adenovirus Serotypes from Subgroups A, C, D, E, and F. *J. Virol.* **1998**, *72*, 7909–7915. [CrossRef] [PubMed]
15. Lenman, A.; Liaci, A.M.; Liu, Y.; Frängsmyr, L.; Frank, M.; Blaum, B.S.; Chai, W.; Podgorski, I.I.; Harrach, B.; Benkő, M.; et al. Polysialic Acid Is a Cellular Receptor for Human Adenovirus 52. *Proc. Natl. Acad. Sci. USA* **2018**, *115*, E4264–E4273. [CrossRef] [PubMed]
16. Podgorski, I.I.; Pantó, L.; Papp, T.; Harrach, B.; Benkö, M. Genome Analysis of Four Old World Monkey Adenoviruses Supports the Proposed Species Classification of Primate Adenoviruses and Reveals Signs of Possible Homologous Recombination. *J. Gen. Virol.* **2016**, *97*, 1604–1614. [CrossRef]
17. Stasiak, A.C.; Stehle, T. Human Adenovirus Binding to Host Cell Receptors: A Structural View. *Med. Microbiol. Immunol.* **2020**, *209*, 325–333. [CrossRef]
18. Ballmann, M.Z.; Raus, S.; Engelhart, R.; Kaján, G.L.; Beqqali, A.; Hadoke, P.W.F.; Van Der Zalm, C.; Papp, T.; John, L.; Khan, S.; et al. Human AdV-20-42-42, a Promising Novel Adenoviral Vector for Gene Therapy and Vaccine Product Development. *J. Virol.* **2021**, *95*, e00387-21. [CrossRef]
19. Shieh, W.-J. Human Adenovirus Infections in Pediatric Population—An Update on Clinico–Pathologic Correlation. *Biomed. J.* **2022**, *45*, 38–49. [CrossRef]
20. Lenaerts, L.; De Clercq, E.; Naesens, L. Clinical Features and Treatment of Adenovirus Infections. *Rev. Med. Virol.* **2008**, *18*, 357–374. [CrossRef]
21. Lopez, S.M.C.; Michaels, M.G.; Green, M. Adenovirus Infection in Pediatric Transplant Recipients: Are Effective Antiviral Agents Coming Our Way? *Curr. Opin. Organ Transplant.* **2018**, *23*, 395–399. [CrossRef]

22. Kuwatsuka, Y.; Atsuta, Y.; Hirakawa, A.; Uchida, N.; Inamoto, Y.; Najima, Y.; Ikegame, K.; Eto, T.; Ozawa, Y.; Ichinohe, T.; et al. Use of Unapproved or Off-Label Drugs in Japan for the Treatment of Graft-versus-Host Disease and Post-Transplant Viral Infection. *Int. J. Hematol.* **2020**, *112*, 841–850. [CrossRef]
23. Uhnoo, I.; Wadell, G.; Svensson, L.; Johansson, M.E. Importance of Enteric Adenoviruses 40 and 41 in Acute Gastroenteritis in Infants and Young Children. *J. Clin. Microbiol.* **1984**, *20*, 365–372. [CrossRef]
24. Kotloff, K.L.; Losonsky, G.A.; Morris, J.G.; Wasserman, S.S.; Singh-Naz, N.; Levine, M.M. Enteric Adenovirus Infection and Childhood Diarrhea: An Epidemiologic Study in Three Clinical Settings. *Pediatrics* **1989**, *84*, 219–225. [CrossRef] [PubMed]
25. Lee, B.; Damon, C.F.; Platts-Mills, J.A. Pediatric Acute Gastroenteritis Associated with Adenovirus 40/41 in Low-Income and Middle-Income Countries. *Curr. Opin. Infect. Dis.* **2020**, *33*, 398–403. [CrossRef] [PubMed]
26. Lu, L.; Zhong, H.; Xu, M.; Su, L.; Cao, L.; Jia, R.; Xu, J. Molecular and Epidemiological Characterization of Human Adenovirus and Classic Human Astrovirus in Children with Acute Diarrhea in Shanghai, 2017–2018. *BMC Infect. Dis.* **2021**, *21*, 713. [CrossRef] [PubMed]
27. Tang, X.; Hu, Y.; Zhong, X.; Xu, H. Molecular Epidemiology of Human Adenovirus, Astrovirus, and Sapovirus Among Outpatient Children With Acute Diarrhea in Chongqing, China, 2017–2019. *Front. Pediatr.* **2022**, *10*, 826600. [CrossRef]
28. Cohen, A.L.; Platts-Mills, J.A.; Nakamura, T.; Operario, D.J.; Antoni, S.; Mwenda, J.M.; Weldegebriel, G.; Rey-Benito, G.; De Oliveira, L.H.; Ortiz, C.; et al. Aetiology and Incidence of Diarrhoea Requiring Hospitalisation in Children under 5 Years of Age in 28 Low-Income and Middle-Income Countries: Findings from the Global Pediatric Diarrhea Surveillance Network. *BMJ Glob. Health* **2022**, *7*, e009548. [CrossRef]
29. Liu, L.; Qian, Y.; Jia, L.; Dong, H.; Deng, L.; Huang, H.; Zhao, L.; Zhu, R. Genetic Diversity and Molecular Evolution of Human Adenovirus Serotype 41 Strains Circulating in Beijing, China, during 2010–2019. *Infect. Genet. Evol.* **2021**, *95*, 105056. [CrossRef]
30. Lambisia, A.W.; Makori, T.O.; Mutunga, M.; Cheruiyot, R.; Murunga, N.; Quick, J.; Githinji, G.; Nokes, D.J.; Houldcroft, C.J.; Agoti, C.N. Genomic Epidemiology of Human Adenovirus F40 and F41 in Coastal Kenya: A Retrospective Hospital-Based Surveillance Study (2013–2022). *Virus Evol.* **2023**, *9*, vead023. [CrossRef]
31. Maes, M.; Khokhar, F.; Wilkinson, S.A.J.; Smith, A.D.; Kovalenko, G.; Dougan, G.; Quick, J.; Loman, N.J.; Baker, S.; Curran, M.D.; et al. Multiplex MinION Sequencing Suggests Enteric Adenovirus F41 Genetic Diversity Comparable to Pre-COVID-19 Era. *Microb. Genom.* **2023**, *9*, 000920. [CrossRef]
32. Carvalho-Costa, F.A.; De Assis, R.M.S.; Fialho, A.M.; Araújo, I.T.; Silva, M.F.; Gómez, M.M.; Andrade, J.S.; Rose, T.L.; Fumian, T.M.; Volotão, E.M.; et al. The Evolving Epidemiology of Rotavirus A Infection in Brazil a Decade after the Introduction of Universal Vaccination with Rotarix®. *BMC Pediatr.* **2019**, *19*, 42. [CrossRef]
33. Do Nascimento, L.G.; Fialho, A.M.; De Andrade, J.D.S.R.; De Assis, R.M.S.; Fumian, T.M. Human Enteric Adenovirus F40/41 as a Major Cause of Acute Gastroenteritis in Children in Brazil, 2018 to 2020. *Sci. Rep.* **2022**, *12*, 11220. [CrossRef]
34. Sarmento, S.K.; De Andrade, J.D.S.R.; Miagostovich, M.P.; Fumian, T.M. Virological and Epidemiological Features of Norovirus Infections in Brazil, 2017–2018. *Viruses* **2021**, *13*, 1724. [CrossRef] [PubMed]
35. Tahmasebi, R.; Luchs, A.; Tardy, K.; Hefford, P.M.; Tinker, R.J.; Eilami, O.; De Padua Milagres, F.A.; Brustulin, R.; Teles, M.D.A.R.; Dos Santos Morais, V.; et al. Viral Gastroenteritis in Tocantins, Brazil: Characterizing the Diversity of Human Adenovirus F through next-Generation Sequencing and Bioinformatics. *J. Gen. Virol.* **2020**, *101*, 1280–1288. [CrossRef] [PubMed]
36. Souza, Y.F.V.P.D.; Souza, E.V.D.; Azevedo, L.S.D.; Medeiros, R.S.; Timenetsky, M.D.C.S.T.; Luchs, A. Enteric Adenovirus Epidemiology from Historical Fecal Samples in Brazil (1998–2005): Pre-Rotavirus Vaccine Era. *Infect. Genet. Evol.* **2021**, *94*, 105007. [CrossRef] [PubMed]
37. Alves, J.C.D.S.; Teixeira, D.M.; Siqueira, J.A.M.; Deus, D.R.D.; Oliveira, D.D.S.; Ferreira, J.L.; Lobo, P.D.S.; Soares, L.D.S.; Tavares, F.N.; Gabbay, Y.B. Epidemiology and Molecular Detection of Human Adenovirus and Non-Polio Enterovirus in Fecal Samples of Children with Acute Gastroenteritis: A Five-Year Surveillance in Northern Brazil. *PLoS ONE* **2024**, *19*, e0296568. [CrossRef]
38. Gutierrez Sanchez, L.H.; Shiau, H.; Baker, J.M.; Saaybi, S.; Buchfellner, M.; Britt, W.; Sanchez, V.; Potter, J.L.; Ingram, L.A.; Kelly, D.; et al. A Case Series of Children with Acute Hepatitis and Human Adenovirus Infection. *N. Engl. J. Med.* **2022**, *387*, 620–630. [CrossRef]
39. Baker, J.M.; Buchfellner, M.; Britt, W.; Sanchez, V.; Potter, J.L.; Ingram, L.A.; Shiau, H.; Sanchez, L.H.G.; Saaybi, S.; Kelly, D.; et al. Acute Hepatitis and Adenovirus Infection Among Children—Alabama, October 2021–February 2022. *MMWR. Morb. Mortal. Wkly. Rep.* **2022**, *71*, 638–640. [CrossRef]
40. Hernroth, B.E.; Conden-Hansson, A.-C.; Rehnstam-Holm, A.-S.; Girones, R.; Allard, A.K. Environmental Factors Influencing Human Viral Pathogens and Their Potential Indicator Organisms in the Blue Mussel, *Mytilus Edulis*: The First Scandinavian Report. *Appl. Environ. Microbiol.* **2002**, *68*, 4523–4533. [CrossRef]
41. Liu, J.; Gratz, J.; Amour, C.; Nshama, R.; Walongo, T.; Maro, A.; Mduma, E.; Platts-Mills, J.; Boisen, N.; Nataro, J.; et al. Optimization of Quantitative PCR Methods for Enteropathogen Detection. *PLoS ONE* **2016**, *11*, e0158199. [CrossRef]

42. Do Nascimento, L.G.; Sarmento, S.K.; Röpke Junior, R.; Fumian, T.M. Evaluation of qPCR for the Selective Detection of Enteric Adenovirus Followed by Sequence-Based Genetic Characterization of F Strains Circulating in Brazil. *Appl. Microbiol.* **2024**, *4*, 1016–1029. [CrossRef]
43. Kageyama, T.; Kojima, S.; Shinohara, M.; Uchida, K.; Fukushi, S.; Hoshino, F.B.; Takeda, N.; Katayama, K. Broadly Reactive and Highly Sensitive Assay for Norwalk-Like Viruses Based on Real-Time Quantitative Reverse Transcription-PCR. *J. Clin. Microbiol.* **2003**, *41*, 1548–1557. [CrossRef]
44. Zeng, S.-Q.; Halkosalo, A.; Salminen, M.; Szakal, E.D.; Puustinen, L.; Vesikari, T. One-Step Quantitative RT-PCR for the Detection of Rotavirus in Acute Gastroenteritis. *J. Virol. Methods* **2008**, *153*, 238–240. [CrossRef] [PubMed]
45. Sarantis, H.; Johnson, G.; Brown, M.; Petric, M.; Tellier, R. Comprehensive Detection and Serotyping of Human Adenoviruses by PCR and Sequencing. *J. Clin. Microbiol.* **2004**, *42*, 3963–3969. [CrossRef] [PubMed]
46. Xu, W.; McDonough, M.C.; Erdman, D.D. Species-Specific Identification of Human Adenoviruses by a Multiplex PCR Assay. *J. Clin. Microbiol.* **2000**, *38*, 4114–4120. [CrossRef] [PubMed]
47. Li, L.; Shimizu, H.; Doan, L.T.P.; Tung, P.G.; Okitsu, S.; Nishio, O.; Suzuki, E.; Seo, J.K.; Kim, K.S.; Müller, W.E.G.; et al. Characterizations of Adenovirus Type 41 Isolates from Children with Acute Gastroenteritis in Japan, Vietnam, and Korea. *J. Clin. Microbiol.* **2004**, *42*, 4032–4039. [CrossRef]
48. Kuraku, S.; Zmasek, C.M.; Nishimura, O.; Katoh, K. aLeaves Facilitates On-Demand Exploration of Metazoan Gene Family Trees on MAFFT Sequence Alignment Server with Enhanced Interactivity. *Nucleic Acids Res.* **2013**, *41*, W22–W28. [CrossRef]
49. Springer. Multiple Sequence Alignment: Methods and Protocols. In *Methods in Molecular Biology*; Katoh, K., Ed.; Springer: New York, NY, USA, 2021; Volume 2231, ISBN 978-1-07-161035-0.
50. Darriba, D.; Taboada, G.L.; Doallo, R.; Posada, D. jModelTest 2: More Models, New Heuristics and Parallel Computing. *Nat. Methods* **2012**, *9*, 772. [CrossRef]
51. Tamura, K.; Nei, M. Estimation of the Number of Nucleotide Substitutions in the Control Region of Mitochondrial DNA in Humans and Chimpanzees. *Mol. Biol. Evol.* **1993**, *10*, 512–526. [CrossRef]
52. Kumar, S.; Stecher, G.; Li, M.; Knyaz, C.; Tamura, K. MEGA X: Molecular Evolutionary Genetics Analysis across Computing Platforms. *Mol. Biol. Evol.* **2018**, *35*, 1547–1549. [CrossRef]
53. Hasegawa, M.; Kishino, H.; Yano, T. Dating of the Human-Ape Splitting by a Molecular Clock of Mitochondrial DNA. *J. Mol. Evol.* **1985**, *22*, 160–174. [CrossRef]
54. Afrad, M.H.; Avzun, T.; Haque, J.; Haque, W.; Hossain, M.E.; Rahman, A.R.; Ahmed, S.; Faruque, A.S.G.; Rahman, M.Z.; Rahman, M. Detection of Enteric- and Non-enteric Adenoviruses in Gastroenteritis Patients, Bangladesh, 2012–2015. *J. Med. Virol.* **2018**, *90*, 677–684. [CrossRef]
55. Kumthip, K.; Khamrin, P.; Ushijima, H.; Maneekarn, N. Enteric and Non-Enteric Adenoviruses Associated with Acute Gastroenteritis in Pediatric Patients in Thailand, 2011 to 2017. *PLoS ONE* **2019**, *14*, e0220263. [CrossRef] [PubMed]
56. Cao, Y.; Yang, J.; Li, N.; Zhang, R.; Jiang, L.; Zhou, X.; Xiang, Y.; Cun, J.; Qiao, E. Detection and Complete Genome Sequence Analysis of Human Adenovirus in Children with Acute Diarrhea in Yunnan, China, 2015–2021. *Arch. Virol.* **2024**, *169*, 34. [CrossRef] [PubMed]
57. Khales, P.; Razizadeh, M.H.; Ghorbani, S.; Moattari, A.; Sarvari, J.; Saadati, H.; Sayyahfar, S.; Salavatiha, Z.; Hasanabad, M.H.; Poortahmasebi, V.; et al. Human Adenoviruses in Children with Gastroenteritis: A Systematic Review and Meta-Analysis. *BMC Infect. Dis.* **2024**, *24*, 478. [CrossRef]
58. Primo, D.; Pacheco, G.T.; Timenetsky, M.D.C.S.T.; Luchs, A. Surveillance and Molecular Characterization of Human Adenovirus in Patients with Acute Gastroenteritis in the Era of Rotavirus Vaccine, Brazil, 2012–2017. *J. Clin. Virol.* **2018**, *109*, 35–40. [CrossRef]
59. Black, R.E.; Perin, J.; Yeung, D.; Rajeev, T.; Miller, J.; Elwood, S.E.; Platts-Mills, J.A. Estimated Global and Regional Causes of Deaths from Diarrhoea in Children Younger than 5 Years during 2000–21: A Systematic Review and Bayesian Multinomial Analysis. *Lancet Glob. Health* **2024**, *12*, e919–e928. [CrossRef]
60. Khan, A.I.; Amin, M.A. Understanding Deaths from Diarrhoea in Children Younger than 5 Years. *Lancet Glob. Health* **2024**, *12*, e891–e892. [CrossRef]
61. Souza, E.V.D.; De Souza, Y.F.V.P.; Medeiros, R.S.; De Azevedo, L.S.; De Queiroz, T.G.A.; Sanz-Duro, R.L.; Marinho, R.D.S.S.; Komninakis, S.V.; Timenetsky, M.D.C.S.T.; Luchs, A. Diversity of Enteric and Non-Enteric Human Adenovirus Strains in Brazil, 2006–2011. *Arch. Virol.* **2021**, *166*, 897–903. [CrossRef]
62. Pratte-Santos, R.; Miagostovich, M.P.; Fumian, T.M.; Maciel, E.L.; Martins, S.A.; Cassini, S.T.; Keller, R. High Prevalence of Enteric Viruses Associated with Acute Gastroenteritis in Pediatric Patients in a Low-income Area in Vitória, Southeastern Brazil. *J. Med. Virol.* **2019**, *91*, 744–750. [CrossRef]
63. Olivares, A.I.O.; Leitão, G.A.A.; Pimenta, Y.C.; Cantelli, C.P.; Fumian, T.M.; Fialho, A.M.; Da Silva E Mouta, S.; Delgado, I.F.; Nordgren, J.; Svensson, L.; et al. Epidemiology of Enteric Virus Infections in Children Living in the Amazon Region. *Int. J. Infect. Dis.* **2021**, *108*, 494–502. [CrossRef]

64. Olsen, S.J.; Winn, A.K.; Budd, A.P.; Prill, M.M.; Steel, J.; Midgley, C.M.; Kniss, K.; Burns, E.; Rowe, T.; Foust, A.; et al. Changes in Influenza and Other Respiratory Virus Activity During the COVID-19 Pandemic—United States, 2020–2021. *MMWR Morb. Mortal. Wkly. Rep.* **2021**, *70*, 1013–1019. [CrossRef]
65. Angoulvant, F.; Ouldali, N.; Yang, D.D.; Filser, M.; Gajdos, V.; Rybak, A.; Guedj, R.; Soussan-Banini, V.; Basmaci, R.; Lefevre-Utile, A.; et al. Coronavirus Disease 2019 Pandemic: Impact Caused by School Closure and National Lockdown on Pediatric Visits and Admissions for Viral and Nonviral Infections—A Time Series Analysis. *Clin. Infect. Dis.* **2021**, *72*, 319–322. [CrossRef] [PubMed]
66. Yeoh, D.K.; Foley, D.A.; Minney-Smith, C.A.; Martin, A.C.; Mace, A.O.; Sikazwe, C.T.; Le, H.; Levy, A.; Blyth, C.C.; Moore, H.C. Impact of Coronavirus Disease 2019 Public Health Measures on Detections of Influenza and Respiratory Syncytial Virus in Children During the 2020 Australian Winter. *Clin. Infect. Dis.* **2021**, *72*, 2199–2202. [CrossRef] [PubMed]
67. Kraay, A.N.M.; Han, P.; Kambhampati, A.K.; Wikswo, M.E.; Mirza, S.A.; Lopman, B.A. Impact of Nonpharmaceutical Interventions for Severe Acute Respiratory Syndrome Coronavirus 2 on Norovirus Outbreaks: An Analysis of Outbreaks Reported By 9 US States. *J. Infect. Dis.* **2021**, *224*, 9–13. [CrossRef] [PubMed]
68. Hayes, L.J.; Uri, H.; Bojkova, D.; Cinatl, J.; Wass, M.N.; Michaelis, M. Impact of the COVID-19 Pandemic on the Circulation of Other Pathogens in England. *J. Med. Virol.* **2023**, *95*, e28401. [CrossRef]
69. Knudsen, P.K.; Lind, A.; Klundby, I.; Dudman, S. The Incidence of Infectious Diseases and Viruses Other than SARS-CoV-2 amongst Hospitalised Children in Oslo, Norway during the Covid-19 Pandemic 2020–2021. *J. Clin. Virol. Plus* **2022**, *2*, 100060. [CrossRef]
70. Yorsaeng, R.; Suntronwong, N.; Thongpan, I.; Chuchaona, W.; Lestari, F.B.; Pasittungkul, S.; Puenpa, J.; Atsawawaranunt, K.; Sharma, C.; Sudhinaraset, N.; et al. The Impact of COVID-19 and Control Measures on Public Health in Thailand, 2020. *PeerJ* **2022**, *10*, e12960. [CrossRef]
71. Maison, N.; Peck, A.; Illi, S.; Meyer-Buehn, M.; Von Mutius, E.; Hübner, J.; Von Both, U. The Rising of Old Foes: Impact of Lockdown Periods on "Non-SARS-CoV-2" Viral Respiratory and Gastrointestinal Infections. *Infection* **2022**, *50*, 519–524. [CrossRef]
72. Grochowska, M.; Ambrożej, D.; Wachnik, A.; Demkow, U.; Podsiadły, E.; Feleszko, W. The Impact of the COVID-19 Pandemic Lockdown on Pediatric Infections—A Single-Center Retrospective Study. *Microorganisms* **2022**, *10*, 178. [CrossRef]
73. La Rosa, G.; Della Libera, S.; Petricca, S.; Iaconelli, M.; Donia, D.; Saccucci, P.; Cenko, F.; Xhelilaj, G.; Divizia, M. Genetic Diversity of Human Adenovirus in Children with Acute Gastroenteritis, Albania, 2013–2015. *BioMed Res. Int.* **2015**, *2015*, 142912. [CrossRef]
74. Qiu, F.; Shen, X.; Li, G.; Zhao, L.; Chen, C.; Duan, S.; Guo, J.; Zhao, M.; Yan, T.; Qi, J.-J.; et al. Adenovirus Associated with Acute Diarrhea: A Case-Control Study. *BMC Infect. Dis.* **2018**, *18*, 450. [CrossRef]
75. Harb, A.; Abraham, S.; Rusdi, B.; Laird, T.; O'Dea, M.; Habib, I. Molecular Detection and Epidemiological Features of Selected Bacterial, Viral, and Parasitic Enteropathogens in Stool Specimens from Children with Acute Diarrhea in Thi-Qar Governorate, Iraq. *Int. J. Environ. Res. Public Health* **2019**, *16*, 1573. [CrossRef] [PubMed]
76. Zhou, J.; Sun, Y. Effect of COVID-19 Protective Measures on the Epidemiology Characteristics of Rotavirus, Adenovirus, and Coinfections among Pediatric Patients with Acute Gastroenteritis in Hangzhou, China. *Microbiol. Spectr.* **2024**, *12*, e04007-23. [CrossRef] [PubMed]
77. Taniuchi, M.; Islam, K.; Sayeed, M.A.; Platts-Mills, J.A.; Islam, M.T.; Khabir, M.I.U.; Rahman, M.; Khan, Z.H.; Begum, Y.A.; Khanam, F.; et al. Etiology of Diarrhea Requiring Hospitalization in Bangladesh by Quantitative Polymerase Chain Reaction, 2014–2018. *Clin. Infect. Dis.* **2021**, *73*, e2493–e2499. [CrossRef]
78. Varghese, T.; Mills, J.A.P.; Revathi, R.; Antoni, S.; Soeters, H.M.; Emmanuel Njambe, T.O.; Houpt, E.R.; Tate, J.E.; Parashar, U.D.; Kang, G. Etiology of Diarrheal Hospitalizations Following Rotavirus Vaccine Implementation and Association of Enteric Pathogens with Malnutrition among Under-Five Children in India. *Gut Pathog.* **2024**, *16*, 22. [CrossRef]
79. Liu, J.; Platts-Mills, J.A.; Juma, J.; Kabir, F.; Nkeze, J.; Okoi, C.; Operario, D.J.; Uddin, J.; Ahmed, S.; Alonso, P.L.; et al. Use of Quantitative Molecular Diagnostic Methods to Identify Causes of Diarrhoea in Children: A Reanalysis of the GEMS Case-Control Study. *Lancet* **2016**, *388*, 1291–1301. [CrossRef]
80. Platts-Mills, J.A.; Liu, J.; Rogawski, E.T.; Kabir, F.; Lertsethtakarn, P.; Siguas, M.; Khan, S.S.; Praharaj, I.; Murei, A.; Nshama, R.; et al. Use of Quantitative Molecular Diagnostic Methods to Assess the Aetiology, Burden, and Clinical Characteristics of Diarrhoea in Children in Low-Resource Settings: A Reanalysis of the MAL-ED Cohort Study. *Lancet Glob. Health* **2018**, *6*, e1309–e1318. [CrossRef]
81. Meier, J.L. Viral Acute Gastroenteritis in Special Populations. *Gastroenterol. Clin. North Am.* **2021**, *50*, 305–322. [CrossRef]
82. Goldar, S.; Rajbongshi, G.; Chamuah, K.; Alam, S.T.; Sharma, A. Occurrence of Viral Gastroenteritis in Children below 5 Years: A Hospital-Based Study from Assam, India. *Indian J. Med. Microbiol.* **2019**, *37*, 415–417. [CrossRef]
83. Borkakoty, B.; Bali, N.K.; Jakaria, A.; Hazarika, R.; Temsu, T.; Gohain, M.; Kaur, H. Norovirus Gastroenteritis in Children Under-Five Years Hospitalized for Diarrhea in Two Cities of Northeast India: A Retrospective Study. *Indian J. Med. Microbiol.* **2023**, *45*, 100397. [CrossRef]

84. Fumian, T.M.; Malta, F.C.; Sarmento, S.K.; Fernandes, S.B.; Negri, C.M.; Belettini, S.A.D.A.; Machado, M.H.; Guimarães, M.A.A.M.; De Assis, R.M.S.; Baduy, G.A.; et al. Acute Gastroenteritis Outbreak Associated with Multiple and Rare Norovirus Genotypes after Storm Events in Santa Catarina, Brazil. *J. Med. Virol.* **2023**, *95*, e29205. [CrossRef]
85. Hassan, F.; Kanwar, N.; Harrison, C.J.; Halasa, N.B.; Chappell, J.D.; Englund, J.A.; Klein, E.J.; Weinberg, G.A.; Szilagyi, P.G.; Moffatt, M.E.; et al. Viral Etiology of Acute Gastroenteritis in <2-Year-Old US Children in the Post–Rotavirus Vaccine Era. *J. Pediatr. Infect. Dis. Soc.* **2019**, *8*, 414–421. [CrossRef]
86. Pabbaraju, K.; Tellier, R.; Pang, X.-L.; Xie, J.; Lee, B.E.; Chui, L.; Zhuo, R.; Vanderkooi, O.G.; Ali, S.; Tarr, P.I.; et al. A Clinical Epidemiology and Molecular Attribution Evaluation of Adenoviruses in Pediatric Acute Gastroenteritis: A Case-Control Study. *J. Clin. Microbiol.* **2020**, *59*, e02287-20. [CrossRef] [PubMed]
87. Pavia, A.T. Viral Infections of the Lower Respiratory Tract: Old Viruses, New Viruses, and the Role of Diagnosis. *Clin. Infect. Dis.* **2011**, *52*, S284–S289. [CrossRef] [PubMed]
88. Kaneko, H.; Suzutani, T.; Aoki, K.; Kitaichi, N.; Ishida, S.; Ishiko, H.; Ohashi, T.; Okamoto, S.; Nakagawa, H.; Hinokuma, R.; et al. Epidemiological and Virological Features of Epidemic Keratoconjunctivitis Due to New Human Adenovirus Type 54 in Japan. *Br. J. Ophthalmol.* **2011**, *95*, 32–36. [CrossRef]
89. Yu, Z.; Zeng, Z.; Zhang, J.; Pan, Y.; Chen, M.; Guo, Y.; Yu, N.; Chodosh, J.; Fu, N.; Che, X.; et al. Fatal Community-Acquired Pneumonia in Children Caused by Re-Emergent Human Adenovirus 7d Associated with Higher Severity of Illness and Fatality Rate. *Sci. Rep.* **2016**, *6*, 37216. [CrossRef]
90. Gopalkrishna, V.; Ganorkar, N.N.; Patil, P.R. Identification and Molecular Characterization of Adenovirus Types (HAdV-8, HAdV-37, HAdV-4, HAdV-3) in an Epidemic of Keratoconjunctivitis Occurred in Pune, Maharashtra, Western India. *J. Med. Virol.* **2016**, *88*, 2100–2105. [CrossRef]
91. Portal, T.M.; Reymão, T.K.A.; Quinderé Neto, G.A.; Fiuza, M.K.D.C.; Teixeira, D.M.; Lima, I.C.G.; Sousa Júnior, E.C.; Bandeira, R.D.S.; De Deus, D.R.; Justino, M.C.A.; et al. Detection and Genotyping of Enteric Viruses in Hospitalized Children with Acute Gastroenteritis in Belém, Brazil: Occurrence of Adenovirus Viremia by Species F, Types 40/41. *J. Med. Virol.* **2019**, *91*, 378–384. [CrossRef]
92. Lun, J.H.; Crosbie, N.D.; White, P.A. Genetic Diversity and Quantification of Human Mastadenoviruses in Wastewater from Sydney and Melbourne, Australia. *Sci. Total Environ.* **2019**, *675*, 305–312. [CrossRef]
93. Blanco, R.; Alcalá, A.C.; Fernández, R.; Ramírez, V.; Rosales, R.E.; Páez, M.G.; Alemán, H.; González, R.; Zerpa, J.; Maldonado, A.J.; et al. Molecular Characterization of Human Adenovirus Causing Infantile Acute Gastroenteritis in Venezuela before and after Rotavirus Vaccine Implementation. *Diagn. Microbiol. Infect. Dis.* **2023**, *107*, 116056. [CrossRef]
94. Chandra, P.; Lo, M.; Mitra, S.; Banerjee, A.; Saha, P.; Okamoto, K.; Deb, A.K.; Ghosh, S.K.; Manna, A.; Dutta, S.; et al. Genetic Characterization and Phylogenetic Variations of Human adenovirus-F Strains Circulating in Eastern India during 2017–2020. *J. Med. Virol.* **2021**, *93*, 6180–6190. [CrossRef]
95. Götting, J.; Cordes, A.K.; Steinbrück, L.; Heim, A. Molecular Phylogeny of Human Adenovirus Type 41 Lineages. *Virus Evol.* **2022**, *8*, veac098. [CrossRef] [PubMed]
96. Hierholzer, J.C. Adenoviruses in the Immunocompromised Host. *Clin. Microbiol. Rev.* **1992**, *5*, 262–274. [CrossRef] [PubMed]
97. Lion, T. Adenovirus Infections in Immunocompetent and Immunocompromised Patients. *Clin. Microbiol. Rev.* **2014**, *27*, 441–462. [CrossRef] [PubMed]
98. Kosulin, K.; Geiger, E.; Vécsei, A.; Huber, W.-D.; Rauch, M.; Brenner, E.; Wrba, F.; Hammer, K.; Innerhofer, A.; Pötschger, U.; et al. Persistence and Reactivation of Human Adenoviruses in the Gastrointestinal Tract. *Clin. Microbiol. Infect.* **2016**, *22*, 381.e1–381.e8. [CrossRef]

MDPI AG
Grosspeteranlage 5
4052 Basel
Switzerland
Tel.: +41 61 683 77 34

Viruses Editorial Office
E-mail: viruses@mdpi.com
www.mdpi.com/journal/viruses

www.ingramcontent.com/pod-product-compliance
Lightning Source LLC
LaVergne TN
LVHW070445061126
851858LV00011B/163
* 9 7 8 3 7 2 5 8 8 3 6 5 3 *